FACING LOVE
ADDICTION

FACING LOVE ADDICTION

*Giving Yourself the Power
to Change the Way You Love*

PIA MELLODY

with ANDREA WELLS MILLER

and J. KEITH MILLER

HarperSanFrancisco
A Division of HarperCollins*Publishers*

HarperCollins books may be purchased for educational, business, or sales
promotional use. For information please write: Special Markets Department,
HarperCollins Publishers, Inc., 10 East 53rd Street, New York, NY 10022.
HarperCollins Web site: http://www.harpercollins.com
HarperCollins®, ▐ ®, and HarperSanFrancisco™ are
trademarks of HarperCollins Publishers, Inc.

Library of Congress Cataloging-in-Publication Data
Mellody, Pia.
Facing love addiction: giving yourself the power to change
the way you love/Pia Mellody with
Andrea Wells Miller and J. Keith Miller.—1st ed.
p. cm.
ISBN 0–06–250604–8 (pbk.: alk. paper)
1. Relationship addiction. I. Miller, Andrea Wells. II. Miller, Keith. III. Title
RC552.R44M45 1992   91–55289
616.86—dc20
05 06 07 RRD(H)   36

To my children,

Jane, Timothy, Benjamin, and Daniel

*each of whose presence helped move me forward in my
recovery journey. My love and concern for them gave me
the motivation to move past my fear and denial
into recovery, and to keep on keeping on.*

—PIA MELLODY

CONTENTS

A NOTE FROM THE AUTHOR

This revised edition of *Facing Love Addiction* includes information I have learned since the first version was published in 1992. First, in the original text I referred to the Love Addict's partner as the "Avoidance Addict." The term "addiction" implies an uncontrollable appetite for the object of desire, and the so-called "Avoidance Addict" displays an opposite trait, a distancing or self-alienation from desire. So it seems sensible to change the term for this partner in a co-addicted relationship to "Love Avoidant."

Secondly, I have learned with greater clarity and detail more about how the interaction between a Love Addict and a Love Avoidant occurs. The dysfunctional cycle of attraction and distancing does not take place unless the dysfunctional energies of both dancers are joined. To think of them separately is inaccurate and misleading in examining the co-addicted relationship.

Third, most of the amended or new material in this edition concerns the nature of the Love Avoidant, who is almost always the product of what I call "enmeshment trauma." In his or her childhood, the Love Avoidant became responsible for the well-being of one of the caregivers, and his or her own well-being became traumatically enmeshed with that of the adult caregiver. I have come to see that as a consequence of this enmeshment trauma, the Love

Avoidant reaches adulthood with at least three erroneous, conscious or unconscious, beliefs.

1. Taking care of needy people brings me self-worth.
2. Taking care of needy people is my job. When I enter a relationship, therefore, it is out of duty and to avoid guilt, not out of love.
3. Getting close to someone means I will be suffocated and controlled, so I avoid closeness.

The new material presented here describes the impact of these erroneous ideas on the emotional cycle of the Love Avoidant.

Fourth, I have modified the way I describe how the Love Addict feels about the distancing behavior or withdrawal of the Love Avoidant. In the original version, I called this distancing "abandonment." Over the years I have come to see that this term is properly applied to relationships between adults and their children. In that relationship the child is helpless to make up for the deprivation of his or her parents' love and physical and spiritual nourishment. In an adult relationship, when we do not get what we want from our partners, we may feel pain. But if we are healthy, we cannot be robbed of our self-esteem or of our ability to care for ourselves. In short, we cannot be abandoned.

I have refined the diagrams of the emotional cyclical stages of the attraction and withdrawal that take place between a Love Addict and a Love Avoidant. I hope these new visualizations will help make the dysfunctional, yet fascinating and dramatic, dance of Addict and Avoidant clearer, thereby making the path to recovery more understandable.

Pia Mellody
Wickenburg, Arizona
2002

PREFACE

This book has been written for those who always seem to choose people to love who apparently cannot or will not "love them back." If you have almost given up on getting a significant other to love you—be it a spouse, lover, child, parent, or friend—we have incredibly good news: Recovery takes serious work, but it is possible. If you are in a love-addicted relationship, you can get into recovery through the treatment approach described in this book.

Love addiction is a very painful compulsive behavior that negatively affects not only Love Addicts but their partners as well. The investigation of love addiction—when one person loves another with compulsive intensity and in ways that are not to the best interest of either person—is a fairly recent phenomenon. In 1975 Stanton Peele and Archie Brodsky wrote a book entitled *Love and Addiction.* But it wasn't until 1986 that another book, *Sex and Love Addicts Anonymous,* by the Augustine Fellowship Staff, ushered in an increasing number of popular books on the subject of love addiction, although few articles or books are listed in the psychological literature.*

---

*See Suggested Reading for some of these titles. We have prepared some brief notes regarding our findings through a psychological literature study, which you can find in Appendix A

It soon became clear to us that what we are calling love addiction has not been separated from the general descriptive concepts and described clearly.

Many people have lumped love addiction in with codependence. In her counseling work, however, Pia Mellody has seen that when certain codependents were apparently successfully treated for their codependence, they still could not relate functionally to or break with the object of their intense desire to enmesh. Evidently, something more was going on.

We are aware that we are jumping ahead of research by describing as clearly as we could what we have gleaned from our own personal and clinical experiences. Nonetheless the therapeutic approach described here has already relieved many people of the painful malady of love-addicted relationships. That fact, and the help we have received in dealing with our own relationships, have encouraged us to write this book.

—Pia Mellody, Andrea Wells Miller, and J. Keith Miller

ACKNOWLEDGMENTS

I wish to acknowledge the contributions of four special people.

First, my friend and mentor Janet Hurley, who is also a therapist. Her loving confrontation and support of my recovery, along with her ideas, helped me face my love addiction and work through it.

Second, my good friend Dr. Ann Worth, who gave me much help and support through my recovery.

Third, my friend Michael Scott, also a therapist, who coined the term "Love Avoidant" to refer to the Love Addict's partner, a term which I used in the first edition of this book. Although in this revised version I now use the term "Love Avoidant," Michael's suggestion was very helpful to me as I first developed these concepts.

And fourth, Dr. Susan Maxwell, Ph.D., who, as my therapist, did what I consider to be a phenomenal piece of work with me. Her talent and support gave me hope that my life and my relationships could and would get better. She made clear and firm interventions on my disease that helped me see what was going on. Working with her is like being on stage in the drama of my life. Like a good director, she gave me ideas about how to deal with the various aspects of the drama and then let me really be myself as I worked out my solutions.

—Pia Mellody

The authors also wish to acknowledge the readers, Vicki Spencer and Ray Thornton, whose careful attention, warm support, and honest feedback helped us write more clearly. Since the responsibility for the final wording and clarification rests with Pia Mellody and ourselves, they cannot be blamed for any remaining mistakes or confusion in the writing.

—Andrea Wells Miller and J. Keith Miller

INTRODUCTION

Katy put down the filmy pink, scented stationery covered with bold, curling handwriting. Her eyes filled with tears, her throat constricted, and she doubled over in pain. "Oh no, Ronnie, not another one!" she sobbed between clenched teeth. "I don't think I can take it again."

The letter, discovered in the pocket of the suit she was preparing for the cleaners, was a love note from Cassie, the young secretary her husband had hired a month ago. It recounted in painful detail the fun-filled rendezvous her husband had kept with the girl—in Acapulco. Katy had thought Ronnie was in San Antonio on business.

Beautiful, tan, and fit, Katy was Ronnie's wife of eight years. At age thirty-five she could easily pass for twenty-five. She had worked hard to keep herself in shape since their near-divorce two years before, and wanted desperately to get her husband's love and attention. But there never seemed to be enough of it.

A few months after they were married, Ronnie became distracted, distant. His business was growing, he said, and he seemed constantly involved in paperwork when he came home. He also had an increasing number of late business meetings and out-of-town trips. Then Katy had learned that Ronnie was having an affair with someone—a stranger she hadn't known. First horrified and then angry, she had confronted him and threatened to leave if he didn't end it. When he had said he needed to think about it, she had actually packed his clothes in boxes, sent them to his office while he was out of town, and changed the locks on the house. She had been terrified that Ronnie would leave, but took action because she was desperate for him to make a decision immediately. If he decided to leave, she already had a plan to fling herself at his feet and get him back, knowing she would feel worthless without him. But she didn't need the second plan.

She had gotten his attention. Ronnie had sent roses, taken her out to dinner, poured out a sensational and sincere apology, and promised he'd learned his lesson. He swore he loved her and never wanted to lose her. She had believed him, and allowed herself to hope and feel happy. The emotional intensity of the near-divorce had rejuvenated her, made her feel alive again, and Ronnie seemed renewed as well. He moved back in, and he and Katy started the long road back to trust.

Katy relied completely on Ronnie for her very being, felt good about herself because Ronnie was back in the relationship, and expected to be cared for and loved the way she knew she needed to be. And after all her efforts to mend the relationship and learn to trust again, she was stunned by the discovery of a new affair.

"What's wrong with me?" she complained to herself. "Haven't I done everything I can to keep him happy? If he left I'd be helpless. I can't balance a checkbook, manage the yard, or schedule car repairs. He knows how much I need him! And he won't talk to me any more. I have no idea what he's thinking or feeling."

On the nights he came home, Ronnie usually grabbed a beer and turned on the six o'clock news. After dinner he'd go to his study and work, or read a novel, or tinker in the garage with some project or other. He and Katy were sexual together two or three times a week, and it was usually satisfying to both of them.

This particular night he noticed Katy's trembling hands and reddened eyes and thought, "Uh-oh, we're going to have an argument if I'm not careful." He braced his shoulders, strode across the living room, and turned on the television set. Halfway through the news a filmy, scented page of stationery floated over his shoulder and landed on his lap. He froze, then remembered leaving the letter in his suit pocket.

Without waiting for a word from Katy he shouted, "Damn it! Why are you such a snoop! I feel like I'm smothering with you lurking around me all the time. I'm getting out of here!" He stormed out and slammed the door, leaving an angry and shaking Katy staring after his retreating back and listening to the sound of the car driving away.

This story could have been about a painful romantic relationship in which no infidelity occurred but other intimacy-destroying conditions existed, or about a mother or father trying to get a teenager on drugs straightened out, or about a devoted son trying unsuccessfully to get his father's attention and love. Or it could have been about a woman continually being hurt by her best friend, who cannot be there for someone who loves and depends on her. These stories all have one thing in common: They describe a very painful addiction to a certain kind of person, a person who is seemingly incapable of responding to single-minded devotion focused on him or her. We call this addictive process "love addiction."

LOVE ADDICTS, THEIR PARTNERS, AND THE RELATIONSHIPS THEY FORM

Facing Love Addiction has three purposes: (1) to describe the Love Addict, the unresponsive person a Love Addict latches on to (whom we shall call the Love Avoidant), and the addictive process created by the two; (2) to describe a recovery process for love addiction; and (3) to describe the characteristics of healthy relationships, and the unrealistic expectations people often have about them. This book is an educational tool as well as a recovery tool; you can use it whether you are a Love Addict or in a relationship with a Love Addict.

First we will examine the characteristics of love addiction and how we distinguish it from basic codependence. We will take a look at the childhood experiences that predispose a person to love addiction. We will look at the emotional cycle a Love Addict experiences when approaching another person and engaging in a relationship. We will examine the progressively more serious frustration, pain, and self-defeating behavior that appears in the later stages of the addictive process. We will also look at the impact of codependent symptoms on the Love Addict's way of relating.

Next we will describe the characteristics of the Love Avoidant, the person to whom the Love Addict is attracted. We will examine the emotional cycle experienced by this person in the relationship with the Love Addict, and we will look at the impact of the Love Avoidant's symptoms of codependence. We will also look at some of the childhood experiences that lead to becoming an Love Avoidant.

Then we will explore the "co-addicted relationship"—the toxic experience these two addict-codependents create when they interact with each other. This relationship seems to be as much an addiction process as alcoholism, drug addiction, or any other addiction, because as the two partners engage in intimate exchanges, they are propelled into obsessive and compulsive behaviors that are not to their best interest, reacting to each other with little, if any self-control, seeing love addiction or co-addicted relationships as distinct from codependence and needing a separate treatment plan in addition to codependence treatment.

The treatment for codependence seems to be a necessary prerequisite to an effective recovery from love addiction. This is because a Love Addict with insufficiently treated symptoms of codependence is virtually unable to recognize the dynamics of love addiction, or to abstain from the addictive parts of the relationship and endure the withdrawal process.

A Recovery Process for Love Addiction

The recovery process that I recommend for the Love Addict has three parts: (1) recovery from love addiction specifically; (2) recovery from codependence to accompany recovery from love addiction; and (3) learning to apply information about the nature of healthy relationships to one's life. In addition, there is information about recovery for the Love Avoidant.

Hardly anyone who experiences a co-addicted relationship has seen a healthy relationship modeled at close range, either by his or her caregivers in childhood or by anyone in adulthood. So Love Addicts and Love Avoidants have little idea how to relate closely and appropriately to someone once they see that their former ways are destructive, abusive, and addictive. We'll describe some characteristics and behaviors of healthy relationships, along with some useful ideas from Pat Mellody about several self-defeating and unrealistic expectations many people have concerning what relationships will be like in recovery.

Pia Mellody

Part I

LOVE ADDICTS AND THEIR RELATIONSHIPS

1.

SEPARATING CODEPENDENCE FROM LOVE ADDICTION

A Love Addict is someone who is dependent on, enmeshed with, and compulsively focused on taking care of another person. While this is often described as codependence, I feel that codependence is a much broader and more fundamental problem area. Although being a codependent can lead some people into love addiction, not all codependents are Love Addicts, as we shall see.

THE DISEASE PROCESS OF CODEPENDENCE

Codependence is a disease of immaturity caused by childhood trauma. Codependents are immature or childish to such a degree that the condition hampers their life. A disease process, according to *Diland's Medical Dictionary,* is "a definite morbid process having a characteristic chain of symptoms. It may affect the whole body or any of the parts, and its etiology (or cause), pathology, and prognosis may be known or unknown." I call the chain of symptoms that characterizes codependence the *core* or *primary* symptoms, and they describe how codependents are unable to be in a healthy relationship with themselves. These are the primary, or core, symptoms of codependence:

1. Difficulty experiencing appropriate levels of self-esteem, that is to say, difficulty loving the self.
2. Difficulty setting functional boundaries with other people, that is to say, difficulty protecting oneself.
3. Difficulty owning one's own reality appropriately, that is to say, difficulty identifying who one is and knowing how to share that appropriately with others.
4. Difficulty addressing interdependently one's adult needs and wants, that is to say, difficulty with self-care.
5. Difficulty experiencing and expressing one's reality in moderation, that is to say, difficulty being appropriate for one's age and various circumstances.[1]

In addition to these, there are also five secondary symptoms that reflect how codependents think other people's behavior is the reason they are unable to be in healthy relationships. The inaccurate thinking represented by these secondary symptoms creates problems in a codependent's relationships with others, but these symptoms stem from the core problem, which is the bruised relationship with the self. These five symptoms are (1) negative control, (2) resentment, (3) impaired spirituality, (4) addictions, or mental or physical illness, and (5) difficulty with intimacy.

1See Pia Mellody, with Andrea Wells Miller and J. Keith Miller, *Facing Codependence* (San Francisco: Harper & Row, 1989), especially chapter 2, for a complete explanation of these symptoms.

1. Negative Control

Codependents either (1) try to control others by telling them who they ought to be so the codependents can be comfortable; or (2) allow others to control the codependents by dictating who they should be to keep others comfortable. Either form of negative control sets up negative responses in the person being controlled, and these negative responses cause the codependents to blame others for their own inability to be internally comfortable with themselves.

2. Resentment

Codependents use resentment as a futile way to try to protect themselves and regain self-esteem. When people are victimized, they experience two things rather intensely: a drop in self-esteem, preciousness, or value, and a profound need to find some way to stop the victimization.

Anger gives people a sense of power and energy. In healthy amounts, anger provides the strength to do what is needed to protect oneself. But when we recycle the anger and combine it with an obsession about punishing the offender or getting revenge, we enter into resentment. Whether or not we actually *carry out* any real punishment or revenge, resentment includes the desire for it. Resentment debilitates the codependent because of the process of replaying the victimization in our minds, which brings on painful emotions such as shame, unexpressed or poorly expressed anger, and depressive frustration. Resentment plays a key part in the way codependents' lives are hampered by blaming others for their own inability to protect themselves with healthy boundaries.

3. Impaired Spirituality

Codependents either make someone else their Higher Power through hate, fear, or worship, or attempt to be another's Higher Power.

Whether or not the codependent is aware that this is happening, this secondary symptom can be quite painful or damaging to the health and functional development of the codependent.

4. Addictions, or Mental or Physical Illness

Our ability to face reality is directly related to our ability to have a healthy relationship with ourself, which means loving the self, protecting the self, identifying the self, caring for the self, and moderating the self. Living out of such a healthy, centered relationship with the self allows us to face the reality of who we are, who others are, who the Higher Power in our lives is, and the reality of our current situation. Developing these abilities and perceptions is the core of recovery from codependence. But when we do not acquire a functional internal relationship and sense of adequacy, the pain that results inside of us and in our relationships with others and with our Higher Power often leads us into an addictive process to alleviate the pain quickly.

I suggest, therefore, that a person with an addiction is probably also a codependent; and conversely, a codependent most likely has one or more addictive or obsessive/compulsive processes. This secondary symptom, then, is the primary link between codependence and any other addiction—particularly love addiction. While experiencing the often unrecognized internal pain of the failure of the relationship with the self, and blaming others for this failure, the Love Addict turns to a certain kind of close relationship, believing the other person can and should soothe the Love Addict's internal pain through giving unconditional love and attention and taking care of the Love Addict.

5. Difficulty with Intimacy

Intimacy involves sharing our own reality and receiving the reality of others without either party judging that reality or trying to change it.

Codependents with the core symptom of difficulty identifying who they are (their reality) and sharing appropriately cannot be intimate in a healthy way, since intimacy means sharing their reality. Without the sharing of healthy intimacy, codependents cannot check out their immature perceptions and they continue to have painful problems in their relationships with others.

WHICH COMES FIRST—RECOVERY FROM ADDICTIONS OR FROM CODEPENDENCE?

Because so many people are codependent and have one or more addictions, the question of which should be dealt with first often arises. It seems to me that powerful addictions that medicate and camouflage reality make it difficult for people to deal with codependence, since codependence recovery involves learning to face reality with increasing maturity.

There seems to be at least four such powerful reality-blurring addictive processes that need to be dealt with (if they are operating in someone's life) *before* a person can effectively deal with codependence. These four addictions are:

- alcohol and drug addiction
- sex addiction
- severe gambling disorder
- severe eating disorders (severe anorexia, bulimia, or overeating) at a near-lethal level

At some point in the recovery process of the core symptoms of codependence, a person's denial about any other addictions, if such addictions are operating, cracks. In some instances, people become aware that they have *switched addictions*. For example, Joe, a recovering alcoholic, may gain forty pounds and realize that instead of beer he is addicted to ice cream. He has developed a food addiction. In other cases, an addiction has been operating all along, but as recovery progresses people become increasingly able to tolerate facing reality (core symptom three) so that the addiction can now be identified. Gwen, for example, who was a recovering anorexic, eventually became aware that she had all too frequently been overdrawn at the bank, charged up to the limit on her credit cards, or in need of frequent loans from friends or parents to help her make ends meet. Gwen's recovery from codependence now allows her to tolerate acknowledging her spending addiction. For whatever reason, people often recognize other addictions that need treatment. Examples of such addictions include:

- love addiction
- eating disorders that aren't lethal at
  the moment (which I call "fat" serenity)
- work addiction
- debting, spending addiction
- religious addiction
- nicotine addiction
- caffeine addiction

LOVE ADDICTS AND THE PARTNERS THEY CHOOSE

Love addiction, therefore, is an addiction that often becomes visible to the codependent only after some work has been done on the core symptoms of codependence. Addressing love addiction can be emotionally very destabilizing because the resistance to facing the denial and delusion around this condition is particularly strong.

The painful patterns of difficulty I have encountered in love addiction are exhibited in relationships made up of two people, each of whom has certain distinct characteristics. One party is *focused on* the partner and the relationship; and the other *tries to avoid* intimate connection within the relationship, usually through some addiction or process that creates intensity. I call the former a Love Addict and the latter a Love Avoidant.[2] The relationship they form I call a co-addicted relationship.

Co-addictions are often husband-wife relationships, but the problem can exist within almost any real or fantasized two-party relationship: parent-child, friend-friend, counselor-client, boss-employee, or a fantasized relationship between an individual and a public figure or popular idol such as Elvis Presley (whom the Love Addict may never have met personally).

A co-addicted relationship is not based on healthy love, but on extreme positive and negative intensity. The Love Addict in particular may experience obsessive and compulsive feelings, thinking, and behavior with regard to the relationship, along with intense emotions including anger, fear, hate, and lust, and so-called love for the other person. In the next chapter we'll examine the characteristics of the Love Addict in more detail.

---

2 When I did an inventory of my past co-addicted relationships, I had the perception that all my partners were fairly consistently walking away from me. All I saw was their backs walking away from me. I devised the term "back-walking-away" in my lectures to refer to the partner who has these characteristics. My friend Michael Scott, also a therapist, coined the term "Avoidance Addict" to refer to the Love Addict's partner, a term which I used in the first edition of this book. Although in this revised version I now use the term "Love Avoidant," Michael's suggestion was very helpful to me as I developed these concepts.

2.

THE CHARACTERISTICS
OF THE LOVE ADDICT

Three characteristics sum up the major behavioral symptoms of a Love Addict.

1. Love Addicts assign a disproportionate amount of time, attention, and "value above themselves" to the person to whom they are addicted, and this focus often has an obsessive quality about it.
2. Love Addicts have unrealistic expectations for unconditional positive regard from the other person in the relationship.
3. Love Addicts neglect to care for or value themselves while they're in the relationship.

Although I see love addiction most often in female partners of sexual-romantic relationships, it is also possible for males to be Love Addicts. A person can also relate as a Love Addict in other kinds of relationships, such as with a parent, one's children, a mother-in-law, a counselor, a close friend, a religious leader, a Twelve-Step sponsor, a guru, or a movie star.

Two Fears: One Conscious, the Other Unconscious

In addition to these three characteristics, Love Addicts are often in the grips of two principal fears. The most conscious fear is the fear of being left. Love Addicts will tolerate almost anything to avoid being left, the fear of which comes from the sorts of childhood experiences described later in this chapter.

The irony is that while Love Addicts want to avoid being left and be connected to someone in a secure way, the close, demanding connection they try to establish is actually enmeshment rather than healthy intimacy—which they also fear, at least unconsciously. This denied fear also comes from the childhood experience of either physical or emotional abandonment, or both. Love Addicts did not experience enough intimacy from their abandoning caregivers to know how to be intimate in a healthy way.

So in adulthood, while Love Addicts often think they are intimate and are seeking an intimate relationship, they are in fact frightened by offers of healthy intimacy because they don't know what to do. When they reach a certain level of closeness, they often panic and do something to create distance between themselves and their partners again.

These two fears—of abandonment and intimacy—bring up the agonizing and self-defeating dilemma of the Love Addict. Love Addicts consciously want intimacy but can't tolerate healthy closeness, so they must unconsciously choose a partner who cannot be intimate in a healthy way.

THE POWER OF ADDICTION: ASSIGNING TOO MUCH TIME AND VALUE

When as recovering codependents we come out of denial about being addicted to a substance or a compulsive behavior, we often realize that our addiction has acquired a control over us that is greater than our own willpower. Whatever we're addicted to initially made us feel better, but eventually begins to make us feel worse. Perhaps the pain of harmful consequences or a confrontation by someone forces us to take a look at what we are doing. We may decide we want to stop using the substance or doing the compulsive behavior, only to find that we cannot. At that point we may painfully realize that we are in the grip of something bigger than we can control, something that has surprisingly strong power over us. In this sense we can say we have, in effect, made this addictive process a Higher Power.

Recovery can begin when we are finally able to say we are powerless over the addictive process and over ourselves in regard to it, and that our lives have become unmanageable. Recognizing and admitting this is the significance of the First Step in any Twelve-Step program.[1]

This process of evaluating an addiction can be applied to love addiction. Possibly the most significant characteristic of love addiction is that we assign too much time and value to another person. Love Addicts focus almost completely on the person to whom they are addicted; they obsessively think about, want to be with, touch, talk to, and listen to their partners, and want to be cared for and treasured by them.

At the beginning this relationship makes Love Addicts feel good.

---

1 We'll see how to write Step One for love addiction in chapter 15.

They admire their partners for, among other things, their evident competence at getting things done, and they rate this person as superior to themselves or as having more power. Along with the perception that the other party has more power comes the tendency to assign  them even more power than they really have, and to expect them therefore to rescue the Love Addicts from the vicissitudes of life, protect them from pain or destruction, take care of and nurture them. When Love Addicts view the other party as having such omnipotent power, they make that person the Higher Power, just as the Higher Power for the alcoholic is the bottle, for the drug addict the drug, for the work addict the work experience.

Eventually, as Love Addicts try harder and harder to manipulate the other person to live up to the mental image they have created— that is, someone who will care for and love them the way they long to be cared for and loved—they experience repeated disappointments, because no one can satisfy these insatiable desires. The relationship then begins to make them feel worse. When the pain gets bad enough, Love Addicts may even decide to end the relationship, only to find that they can live neither with nor without their partners.

Not only do Love Addicts have inaccurate beliefs about who their partner is, they feel angry because of their repeated disappointment in the partner for not behaving according to their expectation (which is of a Higher Power). Love Addicts begin to retaliate with toxic fighting against what they interpret as a willful failure to love on the part of the other party.

While many assume that a codependent is someone who is dependent on, enmeshed with, and takes too much care of someone else, this condition is actually more properly called love addiction. Not all codependents make other people their Higher Power. Some wall themselves off from people; others offend and control without trying to be intimate. Making another person our Higher Power is, I believe, the heart of love addiction, an addictive process of its own.

In order to enter recovery from either codependence or love addiction and stay there, we need to develop a relationship with an appropriate Higher Power a power greater than ourselves that is not another human being, a Higher Power that can provide guidance, solace, and serenity. In the framework of a Twelve-Step program, spiritual development connects us to something that truly has more power than we do so that we get the help we need to offset our own imperfection, fallibility, and lack of power to change. We also get help with the internal struggles all people have with respect to the ordinary difficulties of living.

UNREALISTIC EXPECTATIONS FOR UNCONDITIONAL POSITIVE REGARD (LOVE)

Another powerful characteristic of love addiction is that Love Addicts expect their partners to give them unconditional positive regard at all times, a reflection of the Love Addict's profound lack of self-esteem. Love Addicts usually have serious doubts about their self-worth, and so they are driven more than others to hope for and seek an experience of unconditional positive regard to heal their wounded self-esteem. Like alcoholics, who seek relief in a bottle, or work addicts, who seek it either in the process of staying busy or in achievement, Love Addicts seek in a relationship enough unconditional positive regard to relieve the pain of extremely low self-esteem (a link to codependence).

The tragedy is that Love Addicts are usually drawn to Love Avoidants, who try to avoid commitment and healthy intimacy and are powerfully focused on addictions such as alcoholism, work, or sex. Love Addicts often wind up taking care of Love Avoidants when

Love Avoidants' lives become unmanageable, but the need to do so makes them angry. Since they cannot tolerate the thought of being alone, they stay in the relationship and take care of things, but their anger usually makes them become very controlling and abusive. They can't leave, because they fear abandonment; but they can't be comfortable staying, because their desire to be rescued, cared for, and protected isn't being satisfied.

NEGLECTING TO CARE FOR AND VALUE THEMSELVES

When Love Addicts get into a co-addicted relationship, they cut back on doing the work of valuing and taking care of themselves. I find that most Love Addicts don't know how to take care of and value themselves very well in any case, since they think their care is someone else's job. So when they start a relationship with someone, they expect this person to value and care for them, and they decrease whatever they were doing for themselves before they started the relationship.

I've heard many female Love Addicts say, "When I'm not in a relationship, I do a pretty good job of taking care of myself. I balance my checkbook, get my car fixed, eat balanced meals, handle most of my problems. I even make most decisions fairly well and feel good about my opinions most of the time. But when I get into a relationship, I really deteriorate."

Not only is it irrational to expect unconditional positive regard from another person, it seems preposterous to expect a person who is trying to avoid intimacy to take care of us. Love Addicts, whose skewed thinking tells them that their partners can give them unconditional positive regard and take care of them, are experiencing a failure in their relationship with themselves (a link to codependence).

CHILDHOOD ABUSE EXPERIENCES
OF THE LOVE ADDICT

I have come to believe that people fall into love addiction because of
the unhealed pain from childhood abandonment, and the feeling
that they cannot be safe in the world without having somebody else
hold them up. They cling to a delusional belief that the other party
has the power to take care of them, affirm them, and somehow make
them complete. They keep trying to get the Love Avoidant to match
their unrealistic mental image, and this insistence creates a great deal
of the toxicity between the two of them.

Love Addicts usually didn't have enough appropriate bonding
with their caregivers, and probably experienced moderate to serious
abandonment or neglect in childhood. Young children feel loved to
the extent that somebody takes care of them. Caring transmits the
message, "You're important, you matter, and you are loved." I believe
that when children do not get enough connection and nurture from
a parent, they experience serious difficulty with self-esteem.

Love Addicts usually experienced much deep pain and sadness
and an acute sense of loss during childhood, because a part of themselves was denied the opportunity to grow properly when their caregivers failed to take care of them. This pain and sadness I call "the
pain of the precious child." It goes very deep and back far beyond
the earliest conscious memories.

As children, Love Addicts experienced enormous fear because
they were helpless to create connection with their caregivers. In counseling they often describe that child-fear as a sense of having a loss of
their own breath, as if their air supply had been cut off and they were
literally dying. They also describe being empty because they weren't
filled with nurture by their caregivers. And because they weren't nurtured for who they were, they had trouble being or liking their natu-

ral selves. In addition many were angry because their needs went unmet, since there are fleeting moments when such children are conscious of the abuse they are experiencing.

This severe degree of separation in childhood, the original neglect or abandonment experience, has an extremely toxic effect on children that extends into adulthood. The original abandonment experience is particularly filled with pain, fear, anger, shame, and emptiness. Because the children have no place to express these emotions, they store them up inside and fire them off years later, when the threat or actual experience of being left in adulthood stimulates the accumulated emotions.

Many of these children have had a limited or brief connection with someone, such as a grandparent, which brought relief from the pain, fear, anger, and emptiness of the abandonment. This may only intensify the problem, however, because it teaches them that it is the process of getting connected with someone that brings relief from the anguish.

Even as children, Love Addicts long to get connected, to belong to someone, to finally feel safe by bonding with people who (they think) will fill their gaping emptiness and banish their feelings of inadequacy. They seek The Person who will relieve the stress of the original abandonment experience. As adults, almost any other person will do: a lover, a parent, a friend, their own children, a counselor, a minister. If the other party isn't powerful, it doesn't matter. The Love Addict will invest this person with enough imaginary power and unconditional love to make the Love Addict whole and deliriously happy.

The Fantasy of a Rescuer Is Born

One way such children may escape the pain of severe abandonment by the parents is to fantasize about being rescued by a hero of some kind. Little girls may imagine a knight in shining armor who has loving feelings for her and who does things that demonstrate this love by connecting with her, finally giving her life meaning and vitality. The fantasy is often very much like the fairy tale Sleeping Beauty, in which Sleeping Beauty lies asleep, out of touch with herself and her surroundings, until the life-giving kiss of Prince Charming awakens her. Children spend so much time in this fantasy world because it creates a state of euphoria. I spent hours as a child daydreaming about my knight in shining armor. If I felt bad I could play out this fantasy in my mind, get high in about ten minutes, and stay there for at least two or three hours. I think that when we put a pleasurable picture in our minds and think about it, we can stimulate an emotional response to it that may lead to the release of endorphins into our system. Endorphins literally relieve emotional pain and create varying degrees of euphoria. Such children come to believe that by connecting with such a hero, they, like Sleeping Beauty, will come alive and be safe and valuable at last.

For male Love Addicts the rescuer is often some version of a supernurturing female; for gay men and lesbians it is another same-sex person. This fantasy becomes more and more ingrained in the subconscious mind as the person grows older. As adults these people continue the search for someone to fulfill their rescuer fantasy.

This concept is reinforced in romance novels, movies, and love songs today, and many men and women are strongly influenced by it. Some people may even reason, "It must be possible to connect this way to such a hero, or else why would there be so many movies, books, and songs about it?" The problem with this line of thought is that the relationships depicted there actually reflect unhealthy relationships based on intensity, delusion, and unrealistic expectations, and not mature, healthy love.

A Built-in Sense of Helplessness or Neglect

When the parent abandons or neglects the child, the child receives the message that "I won't care for you because you are worthless."

Abandoned children can't get nurture and affirmation from outside because their caregiver deserts them; and they can't nurture and affirm themselves because they are too immature and no one has taught them what healthy nurture is. So almost all Love Addicts enter adult relationships with a built-in sense of defectiveness and worthlessness and the belief that they are helpless to care for themselves, which comes directly out of the original abandonment by the parent. Accompanying this is usually a fantasy delusion that a white knight of some sort will rescue the Love Addict and fulfill the exaggerated longing created by the abandonment. American culture compounds the problem by promoting this concept, especially by supporting women to believe it.

Also, another effect of the neglect or abandonment on Love Addicts is the belief that in a relationship, if they do not get close enough they will die. This promotes the Love Addict's boundaryless behavior in the co-addictive relationship, which feels like suffocation to Love Avoidants.

THE DISTINCTION BETWEEN LOVE ADDICTION AND CODEPENDENCE

Our notions about how to live life come from our connection with caregivers. Abandonment experiences leave children with the message of worthlessness, as well as with a distorted sense of how to care appropriately for themselves. When a child's natural characteristics are not nurtured, the child develops dysfunctional coping behaviors that illustrate the five primary adult symptoms of codependence cited in chapter 1. Abandoning and abusive behaviors develop because the caregivers did not give appropriate help to their children with regard to life's basic issues regarding self-nurture and healthy interpersonal relating skills.

The first and fourth core symptoms are especially prevalent in Love Addicts: low self-esteem and inability to properly care for the self.[2] The third core symptom, which relates to distorted thinking about reality (who the other party is), is also involved; the other two symptoms are also apparent, though they are less prominent.

When the pain of codependence gets too intense, many of us turn to an addiction to medicate the pain because we do not know any other way to get relief. We find a substance, compulsive behavior, or person to soothe the pain caused by our inability to be in a healthy relationship with ourselves. If the substance, compulsive behavior, or person does a good job, we keep the process going, even though harmful consequences occur more and more often. Eventually we become addicted to the substance, person, or compulsive behavior. The function of an addiction is to remove intolerable reality.

It is often said that we are either addicts or codependents; but I believe that most of us are addict-codependents, experiencing addictions to relieve the pain of our untreated codependence. When we enter relationships, some of us are likely to do so as Love Addicts seeking to calm the pain arising from the root problem: untreated symptoms of codependence. We wind up with relationships that are painful, but that are almost impossible to leave because they do relieve some of the pain of emptiness.

Compulsive behavior is therefore related to addiction, while the pain and stress that a person is trying to remove comes from co-dependence. I often find codependents using alcohol, food, drugs, religion, gambling, work, or relationships to try to remove such pain and stress.

So, not all codependents are Love Addicts. Love Addicts turn to

---

2For more details about the core symptoms, the secondary ones, and how they are set up by childhood experiences, see Pia Mellody, with Andrea Wells Miller and J. Keith Miller, *Facing Codependence* (San Francisco: Harper & Row, 1989), especially chapters 2 and 3.

a person and to compulsive behavior within a relationship as a drug of choice for removing the pain of the difficulties in their relationship with themselves, as defined by the core symptoms of codependence. Other codependents try to soothe their pain through other forms of addictive behavior, and so they are termed alcoholics, compulsive overeaters, anorexics, sex addicts, religious addicts, workaholics, and so on.

Codependence precludes healthy self-love, and those who are compulsively driven to try to get someone else to tell them that they are lovable and loved are termed Love Addicts. The belief of Love Addicts that the other party can and will take care of them comes from the third and fourth adult symptoms of codependence: difficulty owning one's reality appropriately and difficulty taking care of one's own needs and wants. On the other hand, the obsession about the other party, constantly thinking about the person, wanting to be with him or her, to make contact with emotionally, physically, every way possible, is part of love addiction.

· 3 ·

THE EMOTIONAL CYCLES
OF THE LOVE ADDICT

Classic Love Addicts move through a cycle of emotional states as they meet someone, try to live out the childhood fantasy of being rescued, live in denial about the inappropriate behavior of their partner, experience frustration and failure because it seems that nothing they do will make it work, try harder, come out of denial about the inappropriate behavior of the partner, begin obsessing and behaving compulsively, then begin all over again to fantasize about the relationship. Each time they cycle through this pattern, the experience becomes more and more toxic to the Love Addict (and to the Love Avoidant, as we shall see later).

THE CYCLES

Figure 1 illustrates this cycle. Read the progression around the wheel in a clockwise direction, as indicated by the numbers.

1. The Love Addict Is Attracted to the Seduction and Apparent "Power" of the Love Avoidant

Love Addicts meet someone attractive to them, usually a person who is very involved in a lot of things and seems to be managing them very well. This person's apparent power is attractive to Love Addicts because, as we have seen, Love Addicts have been set up to believe they are unable to take care of themselves and are looking for someone who can do the job. Also, if the person is a Love Avoidant he will be behind a wall of seduction, which makes the Love Addict feel special. The Love Addict's need to feel loved then gets triggered.

Often people who are attracted into addictive relationships talk about "love at first sight." I believe we should be cautious when we are experiencing love at first sight; it may really be "addiction at first sight."

2. The Love Addict Feels High as the Fantasy Is Triggered

When Love Addicts begin to develop a relationship with this apparently powerful Love Avoidant, their minds rebound back to the fantasy they developed in childhood about the rescuer. For a woman the rescuer is some form of the "knight in shining armor" who has loving feelings for her. For a man the other party appears to be a "superfemale" who has loving feelings for him.

In either case the selected rescuer also demonstrates this love by an initial and usually intense connection with the Love Addict, which finally gives meaning and vitality to the Love Addict's life. Love Addicts do not see who the other party really is, but instead see the image they created in childhood. They focus on this fantasy image, which they placed like a beautiful mask over the head of the real human being. Love Addicts assign to their partners all the qualities of their childhood fantasy rescuers. Ignoring their partner's reality, good qualities and bad, Love Addicts truly believe that their partners have the fantasy rescuer's attributes and will soon create a wonderful life of wall-to-wall loving and caring.

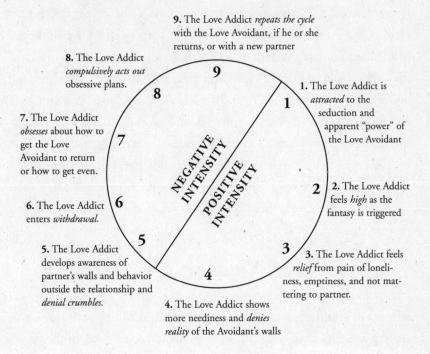

9. The Love Addict *repeats the cycle* with the Love Avoidant, if he or she returns, or with a new partner

8. The Love Addict *compulsively acts out* obsessive plans.

1. The Love Addict is *attracted* to the seduction and apparent "power" of the Love Avoidant

7. The Love Addict *obsesses* about how to get the Love Avoidant to return or how to get even.

2. The Love Addict feels *high* as the fantasy is triggered

6. The Love Addict enters *withdrawal.*

3. The Love Addict feels *relief* from pain of loneliness, emptiness, and not mattering to partner.

5. The Love Addict develops awareness of partner's walls and behavior outside the relationship and *denial crumbles.*

4. The Love Addict shows more neediness and *denies reality* of the Avoidant's walls

NEGATIVE INTENSITY   POSITIVE INTENSITY

Figure 1. The Emotional Cyle of the Love Addict

Even though Love Addicts perceive Love Avoidants to be very powerful, in reality they are not. As we shall see in the next chapter, these chosen partners are also addict-codependents who avoid intimacy through their addictions. But this reality is not clear to the Love Addict.

Instead of developing mature intimacy, Love Addicts seek to enmesh, to merge, to get completely connected to their partners. It could hardly be any other way because the needs of Love Addicts are immense, created by their painful abandonment in childhood.

One of the most interesting facets of love addiction is the way Love Addicts try so hard to get their partners to feel and do the things that match the fantasy they had held in mind for so long, and the intensity of the resulting frustration or anger they feel when their partners do not match it. As a Love Addict, I had an incredible ability to see what I wanted and not see what was actually there. I had this *idea* of who my partner was going to be as our relationship unfolded, and I was determined that he would be that way. This is the honeymoon phase for the Love Addict. Some people call this "romance addiction."

As Love Addicts play out their fantasies in their minds, they experience a wonderful emotional, physical, and mental high. If the relationship is a sexual-romantic one, for example, the sex may be wonderful. Love Addicts now enjoy romantic thoughts and interludes similar to the euphoric state they felt in childhood, when they first developed the fantasy and used it to escape the intolerable reality of their original abandonment.

3. *The Love Addict Feels* Relief *from the Pain*

Experiencing the high from playing out the fantasy in their minds relieves the pain of the reality of being left along, feeling empty, and not being "loved" by the partner in the way they want to be "loved." As relief comes, Love Addicts create more fantasy and begin to feel valued, complete, and full. Love Addicts believe they have really found the person so long dreamed of: the person who will rescue them from their inability to care for themselves, from their loneliness, emptiness, and lack of self-love, and from their inability to feel safe in the world without someone to protect them. Love Addicts believe they have finally found The Relationship that will make them feel whole.

This process, often called "romance," is quite prevalent in our society. In reality the person on whom Love Addicts impose this fantasy is not capable of fulfilling the fantasy at all, but emotionally and/or physically abandons the Love Addict and focuses on an addiction outside the relationship.

4. The Love Addict Shows More Neediness and Denies Reality of the Avoidant's Walls

As Love Addicts feel safer, they begin to show more neediness; but as this neediness appears, Love Avoidants walk away faster, leaving more and more noticeable clues that they are trying to get distance from the Love Addict. Even as Love Addicts gain increasing information about the Love Avoidant's preoccupation with putting distance between them, they ignore or deny the fact that their partner is not present for them in the relationship. By means of this denial, Love Addicts can avoid the agony of rejection. They overlook or minimize obvious signs and excuse the behavior of the Love Avoidant.

"He's so busy right now because it's the fall sales season," a wife thinks, forgetting that her husband was gone just as much in the winter, spring, and summer seasons.

"He deserves to have some time with his friends at the bar after work," a mother says; but in reality her adult son stays out "with the guys" until at least past dinnertime every day and sometimes all night. If he does come home, he may fall asleep in front of the television set or in the bed.

5. The Love Addict Develops Awareness of Partner's Walls and Behavior Outside the Relationship as Denial Crumbles

Eventually Love Addicts begin to have evidence of behavior outside the relationship that becomes increasingly hard to deny because the Love Avoidants are now flagrantly running away from them. Eventually the reality of this behavior becomes clear to the Love Addict, and the fantasy and denial both begin to crumble.

Now the Love Addicts' tolerance of the distancing behavior declines. When the pain gets more intense, Love Addicts earnestly begin to try to control their partners, and threats come out. The intensity escalates and may become very much like the exciting action-packed movies or TV soaps that many of us like to see but pretend we're not in.

At this point, when Love Addicts realize that something or someone else is more important to the partners than their relationship, their fantasy shifts to a nightmare. Now the image of the person who first abandoned them in childhood—a parent or caregiver—comes to mind. They mentally shift from focusing on the make-believe rescuer image and begin to focus on the image of the original abandoner. They still do not see who their partner is, but now assign this person the attributes of their abandoning childhood caregiver.

Out of the resulting pain, anger, fear, and emptiness, Love Addicts may resort to extreme measures to try to bargain with or threaten (somehow to control) their partners and prevent both the continuation of the emotional distancing and the actual physical abandoning of the relationship. Love Addicts experience an obsessive need to know where their partners are going and what they are doing all the time. If their partners don't tell them, Love Addicts often use other methods, such as following the partner, patrolling places they think the partner might be, or calling people and asking about the partner. Other Love Addicts experience the obsessive need to know but endure it silently.

Love Addicts may rage and get hysterical. They may start telling everybody about being "abandoned" in an effort to get somebody to stop the Love Avoidant. They might even talk to their partner's boss. Sometimes they may resort to telling people they meet at the grocery store about the Love Avoidant's behavior, or even announcing it in church. During this part of the cycle, Love Addicts often manipulate extensively, which constitutes attempts at indirect control. They might start doing one or more of the following: dressing seductively, going on vacations with the partner, trying geographical cures (moving to a new town or neighborhood in an effort to "start over," thinking that this will cure the problem), having affairs, trying to get their partners interested by abandoning themselves or displaying extreme neediness. Love Addicts do almost anything they can think of to get the behavior of the Love Avoidant under control; and since almost all the coping methods they learned as an abandoned child are dysfunctional, abusive, and self-defeating, the relationship becomes more and more toxic.

6. *The Love Addict Enters* Withdrawal

Love Addicts finally accept the fact that their partners have abandoned them for someone or something else. In other words, they fully recognize at last that there is something going on in the other party's life that is more important than being in a relationship with them. The Love Addicts' "drug" (the partner) is now withdrawn, and they are intensely aware of the reality of the partner's absence. At this point Love Addicts move into withdrawal, just as any other addict goes into withdrawal when the addictive substance is removed. Withdrawal from an addiction to a person is an intense emotional experience, including pain, fear, sometimes anger, or some combination of these. This is another way in which love addiction can be distinguished from codependence. While the cessation of an addictive process creates withdrawal, recovery from codependence does not. It is also useful to realize that the Love Avoidant, who is not addicted to a person, does not usually experience intense emotions of withdrawal when the relationship ends. He or she is still bent on trying to avoid the intimacy of the relationship.

Now the Love Addicts' original feelings of childhood abandonment are activated along with adult feelings about the current experience of being left. As the intense emotions of pain, fear, anger, and emptiness from the original childhood abandonment combine with adult pain, fear, anger, jealousy, and emptiness about what is going on in their life now, Love Addicts may feel overwhelmed.

This combination of old and current emotions is not as manageable as current adult emotions by themselves might be. A person can tolerate powerful adult feelings, or can handle reexperiencing childhood feelings as they are released in therapy. But the combination of the two can be crushing. This combined pain is extremely intense, and can trigger experiences ranging from feeling depressed to feeling suicidal. The fear can range from anxiety to panic. The anger can range from frustration to feeling rageful and perhaps homicidal. If the Love Avoidant is a sex addict and turns to another lover, the Love Addict's anger, combined with shame carried from childhood, can erupt in the form of jealousy accompanied by a tremendous need to get even.

This experience is devastating when the Love Avoidant leaves, because Love Addicts now face two factors: (1) intense emotional reality and very stark physical losses, such as loss of income, loss of house and other material possessions, loss of a second parent for the children; and (2) all the childhood feelings from the original experience of abandonment and neglect that have accumulated are ready to fire off when stimulated by the experience of being left in adulthood.

The experience of withdrawal from love addiction can be very serious and so intense that many people cannot endure it long enough to get into recovery. Many Love Addicts need help and support from outside themselves. A therapist, a support group, a Twelve-Step program can all be helpful sources of such help and support.

Many Love Addicts who have brought themselves into reality for a brief moment and glimpsed the devastating nature of the withdrawal experience often retreat back into denial rather than face reality and fully enter withdrawal. Many others who enter withdrawal and get overwhelmed by the experience immediately jump into the next point in the cycle, obsessing. This pulls them out of touch with their painful feelings because they stay focused on their obsessive thoughts.

7. *The Love Addict* Obsesses *About How to Get the Love Avoidant to Return or How to Get Even*

Love Addiction, like other addictive processes, is an obsessive-compulsive process used to relieve or medicate intolerable reality. At this stage of the cycle, Love Addicts change the focus of their obsession from the fantasy image of a rescuing hero to either getting the partner back or getting even. Caught in the throes of emotional withdrawal pains, they become obsessive planners. They stay busy planning, which reduces the intensity of the emotional withdrawal. *Whenever* Love Addicts are involved in obsessing, they are not experiencing the full reality of what is happening to them.

If the pain is the greatest feeling, Love Addicts may start obsessively planning how to get relief from the pain, usually through a secondary addiction. They might start planning to get sexual with somebody else (which might indicate a possible sex addiction), create a new relationship and get addicted to that person, turn to the children and get addicted to one or more of them as a Love Addict, get drunk (which might indicate alcoholism), go on an eating binge (which might indicate a food addiction), or go on a spending spree (which might indicate a spending addiction).

For example, Albert felt intense pain after his roommate, Todd, ended their relationship and moved out. He sat alone one evening wearing a comfortable sweatsuit, mindlessly watching television. The thought of eating a bowl of ice cream entered his mind, and the image of a luscious bowl of chocolate ice cream shimmered delightfully before his mind's eye. He had difficulty following the plot of the television show because of his growing obsession about eating the ice cream.

If fear is the greatest feeling, Love Addicts may start planning how to get the Love Avoidant to return. Planning to get the person back seems absurd on the surface. But the reason Love Addicts want their partners back is because Love Avoidants can have a very charming, friendly, sensitive side to their personality, which is usually a large part of what attracted the Love Addict in the first place.

Alice, for instance, couldn't sleep because of her anxiety about being alone. Her boyfriend, Frank, had been gone only three days, and Alice was feeling pretty washed out and very lonely. This particular night she remembered an earlier time in their dating when she had mailed Frank a provocative note—in which she included a pair of panties—asking him to meet her at a certain restaurant. She imagines his reaction if he were to get another note from her now, and spends a lot of time obsessing about sending him such a note and playing out his possible positive reaction in her mind.

Gwen's fear of being alone prompted a slightly different obsession. She found out where Gary's new girlfriend lived and that he visited her almost every night. Gwen started to obsess about taking both children, driving over, and knocking on the door. In her mind's eye she sees the girlfriend open the door, and rehearses speeches where she begs him to come home, thinking that the sight of his two children and herself compared to the tiny apartment and the girlfriend would make him come back home.

Ida, a widow age fifty-five, has been told by her thirty-year-old son, Bob, that he is going to get married and move to a nearby town to start a new job and won't be seeing her as often. He ignored her negative comments about his bride-to-be and made his own decision. In her fear of being on her own without her son's constant caregiving, she obsesses about ways to lure him into staying near her; her obsessions include being helpless about hiring the right roofer to roof the house, replacing her five-year-old car, and so on, instead of learning to do these things for herself or asking for advice from experienced friends.

Paula's fear of being alone after her best friend and roommate has walked out prompts this scenario: She imagines counting up how many sleeping pills she has in the bathroom, swallowing some of them, then calling Nancy and telling her what she's done. She can imagine Nancy rushing back, driving Paula to the hospital, and waiting in anguish to find out if she survives.

If the anger and jealousy are the strongest emotions, Love Addicts often plan how to get even. This can range from creating discomfort for the Love Avoidant (and any playmate involved), to more extreme actions involving destruction of personal property or even bodily damage.

Sylvia planned a relatively mild form of revenge. She imagined how Charlie's face would look if he came back to the house to pack and found his side of the closet stripped and bare.

Tina's obsession wasn't quite so moderate. After her husband, a prominent businessman in their town, had left her, she obsessed about driving into the parking lot of a nightclub where he often went at night and bashing his new Mercedes to a crinkled pulp with a sledge hammer.

8. *The Love Addict* Compulsively Acts Out *Obsessive Plans*

After the obsessive planning phase, Love Addicts usually compulsively act out one or more of the plans they made. They may either run away from the relationship and initiate the same cycle with somebody else, or they may get the Love Avoidant to return and repeat the same cycle with the same person.

Albert carried out his plan by putting on his sneakers, grabbing his billfold, and driving to the grocery store—at two o'clock in the morning. Keeping his head down to avoid seeing anyone, he picked out three flavors of ice cream, four bags of cookies, and several cartons of soft drinks. When he got to the only checkout lane that was open, he saw that there were three other customers ahead of him—all overweight people in sweatsuits with carts full of junk food. Albert planned and carried out an eating binge to take the edge off his pain about Todd's absence.

Alice carried out her plan by writing out the provocative note, buying a new pair of sexy bikini panties, tucking them in the envelope, and mailing it to Frank. Three days later she went to the restaurant at the appointed time—hair done perfectly, nails newly polished, a new dress, perfumed exquisitely. When Frank showed up she begged him to come back, and he melted and returned. Alice reduced her fear of being alone by making and then carrying out a plan to get Frank back. The obsessive planning and compulsive action reduced her fear—even during the three days she waited for their rendezvous at the restaurant. She was in the compulsive-obsessive stage of the addictive cycle.

Gwen finally got the kids into the car, drove over to her ex-husband's girlfriend's apartment, and knocked on the door. When the girlfriend opened the door, Gwen blurted out, "Tommy wants to tell his daddy about his loose tooth!" Her fear of being alone drove her to behave in this extreme manner.

Ida's and Paula's fear also moved them into the compulsive part of the emotional cycle. Ida began bombarding her son, Bob, with her helplessness about the roof, the new car, and countless other things. Paula took some sleeping pills and called Nancy for help.

A week after Sylvia's husband had gone, she carried out her plan by cleaning out Charlie's side of the closet and giving all the clothes to Goodwill before he could come back and get them. Her anger and jealousy prompted her to plan and then carry out this plot designed to create discomfort for her husband.

Tina's anger and jealousy actually drove her to get a sledge hammer, drive to the parking lot, and bash her husband's Mercedes. She was arrested for destruction of private property, and the story was a sensation in the news in that town the next day.

Shannon's anger and jealousy led to an extreme form of revenge. Shannon's husband left and filed for divorce. A few months later he went on a vacation with another woman. While he was gone Shannon took their two small children, broke into his apartment, shot the two children, then shot herself. This is an excessively violent response, of course, and most Love Addicts are not driven this far; but the withdrawal experience of severe Love Addiction can drive someone seeking revenge to extreme measures.

PROGRESSIVE STAGES OF LOVE ADDICTION

I have seen several behaviors in Love Addicts I have counseled that are similar to those of people who have other addictions. They are worth examining in detail.

1. Increasing Tolerance of Inappropriate Behavior from Others

As the fantasy begins to wear off, Love Addicts desperately continue to deny the growing evidence that their partner is excluding them with walls. Their ability to tolerate and ignore flagrant signs of distancing increases.

For example, let's say Marianne, a Love Addict in this stage, comes to see her counselor. The counselor might say, "Well, how was it this week?"

"Well, he only smacked me three times, but it wasn't that bad, I didn't get any bruises or anything."

The counselor is dismayed, observing the increased tolerance of inappropriate behavior. Marianne comes back for her next session, and the counselor asks how this week went.

"Well, he slapped me about six times, but I only got one black eye. So I guess it wasn't so terrible." This is increasing tolerance.

It could also be a man increasingly tolerating the inappropriate behavior of a female Love Avoidant. Perhaps he says, "She stayed out all night only once this week."

2. Greater Dependence on the Person

Love Addicts surrender more and more of their responsibility for daily tasks of the relationship to the other party. More and more of the Love Addict's needs and wants become the responsibility of the partner.

For example, Sandra gave her husband, Paul, the trust papers to her inherited family estate, saying, "Paul, you handle this for me. You're smart. I know you can handle it better than I can." Angie requires her daughter, Mabel, to take the clothes to the cleaners, saying that she forgets which day the special price is offered. Joe insists that his close friend, Max, be the one to call and set up their lunch appointments, saying that he just can't remember where Max's phone number is.

3. Decrease in Self-care

Love Addicts, who at one time dress nicely and take care of their personal grooming, may begin to show a greater state of dishevelment each time they come to see their counselor. For example, Fred, who had a neatly trimmed mustache and medium-length hair, came to his therapy group with increasingly longer and shaggier hair. His mustache began to cover his top lip and soak up coffee as he sipped it. Maureen, usually attractively dressed in skirts and blouses, began to show up in baggy sweatsuits, and she, too, stopped getting her hair cut or styled.

4. Numbness to Feelings

Love Addicts continue to experience waves of pain, anger, fear, shame, and jealousy. Yet, when they talk to their counselors, they report being numb to those feelings.

5. Feeling Trapped (or Stymied)

If some kind of relief doesn't come, Love Addicts may enter the final stages of the addiction: an overpowering sense of being stymied and helpless to fix the relationship, or to escape the pain by ending it. Reality becomes even more overwhelming because Love Addicts have lost the ability to care for and value themselves. If Love Addicts enter this stage and begin to feel stymied, they also may experience increasing despair, disillusionment, and depression. Their behavior can become bizarre and inappropriate. Along with the feeling of being trapped, they may experience a loss of power that leads to a loss of the ability to respond to what is happening.

6. The Final Stages

As Love Addicts progress through the stages of the illness, they feel abused by their partners. At the same time, however, they are abusive *toward* their partners. One form of abuse is the inability to see the ways in which the other person *is* able to be there for them and occasions on which the partner's behavior is connecting rather than distancing. Instead Love Addicts see almost everything the other person does in a negative light. For example, the partner may compliment the Love Addict, which is one way to be present for someone. When Love Addicts interpret this through their own negative filter, they cannot hear the compliment. Their partner might say, "You really did a good job on your garden this year." And the Love Addict may respond, "Well, it's not really the way I wanted it. Last year's garden was better," and get so focused on feeling inadequate that they miss the compliment.

A Love Addict's demand to be loved in spite of the impact of immature, irrational, offensive behavior toward the Love Avoidant is one way the Love Addict abuses the Love Avoidant. It's unreasonable to expect to be loved unconditionally, especially when one is acting inappropriately toward the other person.

Love Addicts also have trouble seeing how difficult they are to live with, because they are focused on how difficult the partner is making their life. They don't see themselves as the addict. They abuse their partners by demanding to enmesh with them and be taken care of, yet they think these are reasonable requests—that in fact it is evidence of love and trust. Love Addicts think that the Love Avoidant's need to get away from them is abnormal, when actually what they are asking for is threatening and more than anyone can give.

Love Addicts enter withdrawal, then obsess about and often carry out some plan of retaliation, but fail to see this behavior as offensive. Threatening or actually attempting suicide, telling the boss all about the gory details of the other party's private life, bashing cars, dragging the children to another woman's apartment and using them as pawns to manipulate the partner, giving away the partner's clothes without permission, raging, getting hysterical—all are examples of offender behavior. As any of these continues, Love Addicts themselves are jettisoning the relationship.

The Partners love Addicts Choose: Characteristics of the Love Avoidant

Love Addicts are attracted to people with certain identifiable and fairly predictable characteristics, and people with these characteristics are attracted to Love Addicts in return. The primary attribute marking all of the characteristics of the "model" partner for a Love Addict is avoidance, which seems incredible to their partners since Love Avoidants come on to their partners so strongly at first.

Characteristics of the Love Avoidant

Love Avoidants have at least three characteristics that combine to result in avoiding intimacy:

1. Love Avoidants evade intensity within the relationship by

creating intensity in activities (usually addictions) outside the relationship.

2. Love Avoidants avoid being known in the relationship in order to protect themselves from engulfment and control by the other person.

3. Love Avoidants avoid intimate contact with their partners, using a variety of processes I call "distancing techniques."

I have seen the Love Avoidant's characteristics most often in the male partner of romantic relationships between a man and a woman, although there are romantic relationships in which the reverse is true. It is also possible for one partner in a gay or lesbian relationship to have the characteristics of a Love Avoidant. In addition, the characteristics of an Love Avoidant can surface during other kinds of relationships— with children, with parents or parents-in-law, with a therapeutic client, or with a close friend, to name just a few possibilities.

A fundamental trait of the relationships Love Avoidants have with others is real abandonment. Love Avoidants don't share who they are in a realistic way with their children. They conduct life from behind protective emotional walls, and, like unseen puppeteers, they continually try to control the choices of other people with whom they are seeking relationship.

Two Fears: One Conscious, the Other Unconscious

Love Avoidants consciously (and greatly) fear intimacy because they believe that they will be drained, engulfed, and controlled by it. As we shall see, in childhood Love Avoidants were drained, engulfed, and controlled by somebody else's neediness, somebody else's reality, somebody else's existence, and they don't want to go through that experience again. This experience of childhood enmeshment created a deeply ingrained conviction that more intimacy will bring more misery, based on experience both with the original caregivers and with other Love Addict partners.

At the same time Love Avoidants fear being left at some level. This fear is usually unconscious, although in some Love Avoidants it is fairly close to the conscious level. The fear in adulthood stems from being abandoned as a child by the caregiver, since when a child is forced to nurture the parent, the parent abandons the child's needs for nurture (this is explained more fully on page 47). Although childhood abandonment is a less obvious experience for Love Avoidants than enmeshment, it is nevertheless real. Since Love Avoidants usually had very little human contact in childhood that relieved the pain, fear, and emptiness of abandonment, they did not learn that a relationship can relieve these feelings. But this unconscious fear of being left draws Love Avoidants toward relationships, even though they have great difficulty making a commitment or connecting to their partner.

At an unconscious level, Love Avoidants recognize and are attracted to the Love Addict's strong fear of being left because Love Avoidants know that all they have to do to trigger their partner's fear is threaten to leave. Love Avoidants believe that being in control this way will allow them to escape being drained, engulfed, and controlled, and at a deeper level to avoid being left themselves.

So Love Avoidants have the same two fears as Love Addicts: intimacy and being left. The difference is that what is conscious for one is unconscious for the other. Love Addicts have a strong fear of abandonment and an unconscious fear of intimacy, which causes them unconsciously to pick someone who can't be intimate. Love Avoidants have a strong fear of intimacy, and yet also a deep underlying fear of being left. This keeps them on the front edge in relationships, where, for part of the time, they can feel powerful by meeting someone's needs without being engulfed.

EVADING INTENSITY WITHIN THE RELATIONSHIP

A major goal for Love Avoidants is to keep intensity within the relationship to a minimum, because relationship intensity feels very draining, is frightening, and threatens to be overwhelming. They avoid intimacy by focusing on something outside the relationship in an addictive way. Any addiction will do, and the effect is the same: They are not available to the partner for an intimate relationship. By focusing on something outside the relationship, Love Avoidants create too much distance from the Love Addict. Their partners get the feeling that Love Avoidants are not really in the relationship because, in a very real way, they are not.

In addition, the intensity of focus outside the relationship gives Love Avoidants a sense of energy, of being involved in life; they don't feel such energy within the relationship because they keep it at a low intensity. A Love Addict's awareness of this absence of energy furthers a sense of too much distance from his or her partner.

AVOIDING BEING KNOWN BY THE PARTNER

As we have seen, intimacy involves sharing information about the self with a nonjudgmental listener. Love Avoidants, when faced with the possibility of intimate contact with another, try to avoid being known by the other. I believe this is because they have an intense fear of being used, engulfed, controlled, or manipulated if they share themselves with someone else. This trait manifests itself in their reluctance to tell their partners what they need or want, requiring their partners to guess these things.

These fears of being used and engulfed, and of being intimate, come to Love Avoidants from their childhoods, in which information they shared was indeed used by their caregivers to manipulate them into taking care of the caregiver. In addition, as we have seen, Love Addicts also seek to enmesh with their partners and be taken care of and loved unconditionally, and they will use personal data about Love Avoidants to this end.

Also, if Love Addicts fail to follow through after being directly asked for help with meeting a need or want, then Love Avoidants feel let down and betrayed, as they were in childhood.

AVOIDING OPPORTUNITIES FOR INTIMATE CONTACT WITHIN THE RELATIONSHIP

Love Avoidants use various distancing techniques to avoid intimacy. These processes include using walls instead of healthy boundaries, keeping some form of distraction going on, using psychological control devices, and engaging in addictive behavior.

Using Walls Instead of Healthy Boundaries

Healthy intimate contact between people comes when one person shares his or her reality with the other, and the other comprehends it without judging or trying to change it. This can happen on one or more of several reality levels: physical, sexual, emotional, and intellectual.[1]

1For a more detailed discussion of intimacy as sharing reality see Pia Mellody, with Andrea Wells Miller and J. Keith Miller, *Facing Codependence* (San Francisco: Harper & Row, 1989), 54–56.

Healthy boundaries are a vital ingredient to such intimate exchanges. They provide protection so that we can be comfortable while hearing someone else's reality, even when we don't like it, or while sharing our own. Boundaries also serve to curb our own reality so that we can express it appropriately and not abuse or violate others with it.[2]

One of the core symptoms that many codependents experience is the inability to maintain healthy boundaries. Some people use walls instead of healthy boundaries. Walls do protect us; but unlike boundaries, they are a barricade to intimacy. It is almost impossible to experience intimacy when one or both people are using walls.

Imagine you are standing on the edge of your lawn, at the property line between your yard and your neighbor's yard. This property line is like a healthy boundary. You know where it is, you can see past it, talk to your neighbor across it, have a relationship over it. But both you and your neighbor know where your own rights begin and end.

If you build a high brick wall or a wooden fence along the property line, then there is a physical obstacle between you and your neighbor. You can no longer see him or talk to him as easily. The wall gives you protection and privacy but interferes with your relationship with your neighbor. While high brick walls may have some advantages with regard to property lines, relationship walls prohibit intimate relationships.

Several kinds of walls hamper our ability to relate to others. Walls of anger and fear, for example, use strong emotions to keep people at a distance. Love Avoidants may also use a wall of silence, which effectively keeps talking to a minimum; a wall of artificial maturity, keeping calm at all times and never showing emotions (an avoidance of

2For a more complete discussion of boundaries see Mellody, Miller, and Miller, *Facing Codependence*, 11–21.

emotional intimacy); and a wall of pleasantness, being courteous at all times, even to the point of withholding information from the partner about difficulties in the relationship—information that might allow the difficulties to be negotiated (avoidance of intellectual and emotional intimacy).

Using Distractions

Another distancing technique that Love Avoidants use is to keep busy with something when in the presence of the partner. Keeping the radio playing while driving in the car is a common example. A Love Avoidant might keep the television going when at home, or stay busy repairing things and tinkering with hobbies. Sometimes Love Avoidants get deeply involved in a sport such as tennis, golf, bowling, or softball, so that they have a reason to spend a lot of time away from the partner. There is nothing wrong with enjoying any of these activities, except when they are done to avoid intimate contact within the relationship. Even when two people participate in the sports together, such as a father and son who play golf or go hunting together, the involvement in the activity can become a substitute for intimate exchange of thoughts and feelings.

Staying in Control of the Relationship

The relationship between value, power, and money in our culture is fascinating. Whenever our sense of value is increased, our sense of power and our ability to make money often rises. By the same token, if we empower ourselves in some way, our sense of value and our ability to make money may increase. Conversely, if our ability to earn money decreases, our sense of value and power also seem to decrease. A change in any one of the three affects the other two in the same direction—up or down.

Love Avoidants try to control the money, be the powerful one, and have more value as a way to be in control of their partners. This

deep need to be in control stems from their greatest fear: that someone else will dictate who they have to be.

At first glance it seems contradictory that a person who works so
hard to avoid being in a relationship also wants to control someone
else into staying in that relationship. What prevents this person from
just going off and being an isolated hermit? I believe it is the underlying fear of being left coupled with the sense of value and empow-
erment that comes from rescuing and being adored by the needy, and
apparently helpless, Love Addict. Love Avoidants want and need to
be in a relationship and to feel connected; but they have to be in a
relationship in a very protected way because they fear being engulfed
or controlled by the relationship. They use the dynamics of value,
power, money, and withholding intimacy to be the one in power and
therefore in control.

Another method of staying in control is to work hard to win or
be right in all situations, because to be wrong is to lose control. Yet
another technique is to avoid arguing, because losing an argument
means facing the inevitable logic of the partner's argument and having to change or admit one made a mistake, thus having a sense of
losing control.

Some Love Avoidants also may use physical power and abuse to
control the Love Addict. This is an important factor in the operation
of many physically abusive relationships.

Addictions

The Love Avoidant's focus on one or more addictions accomplishes
several purposes. The primary one is to create intensity outside the
relationship in order to put energy and interest in the life of the Love
Avoidant. A second purpose is to medicate the intolerable reality that
Love Avoidants are not equipped to face. A third purpose is to get the
attention of the Love Addict. The message to the Love Addict is,
"There is something more important than you are in my life." This

keeps the challenge of "winning" the Love Avoidant's heart in the center of the Love Addict's attention. And fourth, Love Avoidants can further control Love Addicts by frightening them with the effects of the addiction.

CHILDHOOD ABUSE EXPERIENCES OF THE LOVE AVOIDANT

It is in our family of origin that we learn how to be in a relationship. The Love Avoidant's family of origin usually had strong connection among the members, but with too much intensity. I call this form of extremely intense connection "enmeshment." While enmeshment is very different from healthy bonding, to the child this enmeshment seems to be healthy.

The Difference Between Enmeshment and Proper Bonding

There is a proper close parent-child relationship called bonding, a functional activity on the part of parent to the child. This emotional connection is like an emotional umbilical cord that goes from the parent to the child so that the parent, rooted in a mature, stable place, nurtures and supports the child.

Enmeshment is the opposite. The emotional connection between parent and child is also like an umbilical cord, except the energy flow is being extracted from the child to nourish the parent. These enmeshed children get drained dry and used by Mom's or Dad's need for companionship, attention, and love. Children who have been in enmeshed relationships with a parent most often become Love Avoidants. (The Love Addict was not used in this smothering way, but was abandoned and left alone.) I believe we must have respect for the plight of Love Avoidants. Their recovery process is not any easier to deal with than that of Love Addicts. In the process of being used by their caregivers, Love Avoidants were also abandoned; because while they were taking care of their parents, no one was there taking care of them.

Emotional Sexual Abuse

Enmeshment is a form of emotional sexual abuse. It happens when parents draw a child into the midst of the adult relationship they are having. Parents who draw their children into their relationship are usually too immature to be intimate with another adult; they find it too threatening and too painful. But they realize they can be intimate with their children because the children (1) are vulnerable and (2) won't abandon them, but must stay near them for survival. So one or both of a Love Avoidant's parents have a relationship with him or her that is more important to this parent than the relationship with the other parent.[3]

As we have seen, Love Addicts contributed to the family by being needless, wantless, quiet, good, isolated, and unconnected—not taking anything from the family. Love Avoidants had similar experiences, but they went a step further. As children they too did not take anything from the family; they also had to provide from their own resources to support or nurture the parents.

Such children get overwhelmed by the intensity created within this enmeshed relationship and by the draining effect it has on them. The double message they get from the enmeshing adult is, "You will be the Higher Power, focused on and having my total devotion. You will be in charge and in control." But the secret unspoken message is, "At the same time you will be drained dry and engulfed by intensity as you emotionally sustain me."

3For more details about emotional sexual abuse, see *Facing Codependence*, 162–69.

Although Love Avoidants (even as children) get to be powerful and in control as they take care of the parent with whom they're enmeshed, they also become responsible for the direction of their parent's life. The person who controls also gets responsibility for how the other person's life is going, and this responsibility for the welfare of an adult creates an overwhelming sense of being drained for the child.

Parents who enmesh with and drain their children are usually Love Addicts. Heterosexual male Love Avoidants have usually experienced enmeshment with their mothers. Many heterosexual women today are Love Addicts in relationships with Love Avoidants, and they experience abandonment by their husbands. These abandoned women often turn to a son and have a relationship that is more important to them than their relationship with their husbands, because their husbands aren't there. This creates another Love Avoidant; for when the son grows up, he is powerfully attracted to other Love Addicts, and enters relationships avoiding intimacy for fear of being engulfed and drained.

I don't want to implicate only men because they abandon their wives; the wives are equally responsible for emotionally and sexually abusing their sons (or daughters, in some cases) instead of facing the problem in their relationship with the husband and doing something about it. Emotional sexual abuse can happen to a woman too. Her father may make her "Daddy's Little Girl," put her on a pedestal, and make her more important than Mom. This is often how women become Love Avoidants.

The Double Bind: Being a Higher Power But Being Engulfed

Love Avoidants can grow up feeling very good about themselves in their role in the family of origin because they see that they must have been quite special to be taking care of one or both parents. They learn that to be connected means they get to be the Higher Power to someone else, and yet it also means to be drained. Such children often come to believe they are better than others, and in an elusive way this belief keeps them deluded about their true level of self-esteem and competency, making them either grandiose or filled with unrealistic feelings of inferiority. They can even believe that a healthy amount of competency and self-esteem is somehow not enough.

In summary, the child who has been enmeshed develops three erroneous relational beliefs:

1. Taking care of needy people brings me self-worth.
2. Taking care of needy people is my job. When I enter a relationship, therefore, it is out of duty and to avoid guilt, not love.
3. Getting close to someone means I will be suffocated and controlled, so I avoid closeness.

Codependence

Love Avoidants are not equipped to form intimate relationships. Because they came out of a family of origin that was less than nurturing, Love Avoidants have symptoms of codependence. Core symptoms number two and three (difficulty with boundaries and difficulty owning and expressing one's reality) are very prevalent in Love Avoidants. They have not been taught how to have healthy boundaries, since their rights and needs were not respected or taken care of by the parents.

The other symptoms of codependence are involved, but to a lesser degree. For example, Love Avoidants usually believe they are better than others, but sometimes swing down to a deep sense of worthlessness. They also lack the ability for proper self-care, although this symptom isn't usually as severe as in the life of Love Addicts. Self-containment is also difficult to varying degrees for Love Avoidants.

Also, Love Avoidants usually have turned to one or more addictions to medicate the pain of being codependent. As we saw in chapter 1, this is a secondary symptom of codependence. So both partners are addict-codependents, each turning to addictions to medicate the pain of their untreated codependence symptoms.

Traits of Each Role Can Be Found in the Same Person

Some people grow up in families in which they experienced enmeshment from one parent and abandonment from the other, or perhaps one parent enmeshed with them for a while, then abandoned them (such as a single mother who enmeshes with her son, then meets a man and develops a relationship with him, abandoning her son). In the family of origin of people who were both enmeshed and abandoned, there was no appropriate emotional bonding between the child and the parent. They learned that to be connected means both to be engulfed and drained and to be abandoned. Therefore they have the capacity to operate out of either set of characteristics, those of a Love Addict or an Love Avoidant.

Such people usually alternate between being a Love Addict and an Love Avoidant. A Love Addict might be abandoned by an Love Avoidant, then say, "Well, nuts to this. I'm never going to get that hooked on anybody again." So this person meets a very needy person and becomes the Love Avoidant in control. Then the person tries to relate that way and finds out that it doesn't work either, and switches once again to the Love Addict role.

Sometimes couples can take turns being the Love Addict and the Love Avoidant, because they both may be sex addicts, work addicts, or alcoholics. Perhaps when the wife is relating as a Love Addict, the husband is a sex addict/Love Avoidant; but when the husband is relating as a Love Addict, the wife becomes an alcoholic/Love

Avoidant. The specific addiction involved for each one doesn't matter. When both people alternate between both roles, it creates the most intense, crazy, often homicidal relationships of all, where a couple may even engage in physical violence as well as emotional and psychological intensity. This is a serious problem for our society.

5

THE EMOTIONAL CYCLES
OF THE LOVE AVOIDANT

Love Avoidants have their own relational cycle, which is just as toxic as that of the Love Addict. They enter relationships more to caretake than to be relational and use walls of seduction to keep from feeling suffocated as they caretake. This caretaking from behind walls breeds resentment in the Love Avoidant because it is draining. The resentment enables them to distance from the relationship where they create intensity which feels good. They eventually feel guilty about the distance and then return to the caretaking or move on to another relationship.

THE CYCLES

Figure 2 is a diagram of this emotional cycle in the form of a wheel. Read this wheel in a counterclockwise direction, as indicated by the numbers.

1. The Love Avoidant Enters Relationship Because He Will Feel Guilty If He Says No.

One of the effects of the trauma of childhood engulfment is that the person being enmeshed learns that to be relational is to caretake, and in that associates being relational with duty. I also think that caretaking of needy people becomes part of the Avoidant's value system, so that if he refuses to caretake, he feels guilty.

2. The Avoidant Attempts to Be Relational Behind a Wall of Seduction to Avoid Feeling Vulnerable and to Make the Partner Feel Loved or Special.

Engulfment causes the Avoidant to associate being rational with suffocation and control, so in order to avoid this, the Avoidant walls in

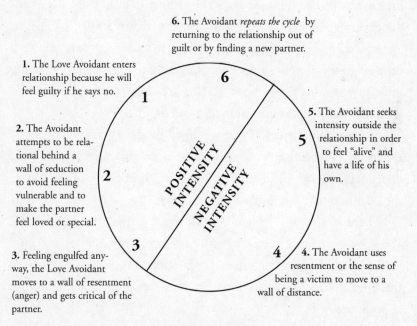

6. The Avoidant *repeats the cycle* by returning to the relationship out of guilt or by finding a new partner.

1. The Love Avoidant enters relationship because he will feel guilty if he says no.

2. The Avoidant attempts to be relational behind a wall of seduction to avoid feeling vulnerable and to make the partner feel loved or special.

3. Feeling engulfed anyway, the Love Avoidant moves to a wall of resentment (anger) and gets critical of the partner.

5. The Avoidant seeks intensity outside the relationship in order to feel "alive" and have a life of his own.

4. The Avoidant uses resentment or the sense of being a victim to move to a wall of distance.

POSITIVE INTENSITY

NEGATIVE INTENSITY

Figure 2. Love Addict Cycle

and manipulates the partner with seduction. The seduction causes the Love Addict partner to feel loved or special, usually to overlook the fact that the Avoidant is actually walled in. Using a wall instead of a boundary, the Avoidant does not tell the partner what is really important to him or her and does not listen to what is important to the partner. So the relationship has the appearance of intimacy without being intimate.

3. Feeling Engulfed Anyway, the Love Avoidant Moves to a Wall of Resentment (Anger) and Gets Critical of the Partner.

Sooner or later Love Avoidants begin to be overwhelmed by the neediness of their Love Addict partner. They begin to feel emotions that come from their old childhood experience of engulfment, which was frightening, painful, and draining - almost as if their very life-breath was being siphoned out. This differs slightly from the abandonment experience of Love Addicts, which was full of pain, fear, anger, and emptiness—the sense of living in a near-vacuum with very little air to breathe. Both have an experience that is similar to having difficulty breathing, but Love Addicts are abandoned and deprived, while Love Avoidants are enmeshed and drained.

As Love Avoidants feel overwhelmed by partners' neediness and intensity, they judge Love Addicts as less-than because of this dependence. Love Avoidants also have a sense of being controlled by the neediness of Love Addicts.

There is also an element of old anger carried from childhood about having to care for the parent. In the current adult relationship, this old anger often comes up and may cause Love Avoidants to judge the Love Addicts' imperfections and neediness more harshly than is appropriate.

4. The Avoidant Uses His Resentment or Sense of Being a Victim of the Relationship to Move to a Wall of Distance.

Resentment is the anger the Avoidant feels because of thinking he or she has been victimized by the partner's neediness or by the partner's "demands" for connection in the relationship. The avoidant feels quite justified to feel resentment because of believing he or she has been injured by the other person.

5. The Avoidant Seeks Intensity Outside the Relationship in Order to Feel "Alive" and Have a Life of His Own.

Enmeshment by a caregiver or parent causes the child to "adapt" to the needy caregiver. In this adaptation, the child has to shut down his spontaneity. He gradually feels more and more empty or dead inside himself or herself and at some point seeks intensity to mask this deadness.

One of the interesting things to note here is that it is in our spontaneity we are most real or alive. That is when we are accessing our Authentic Selves, which is where our spiritual reality resides. Therefore, the spontaneity that allows us to be real allows us to be spiritual. It is in contact with this energy that our lives have real meaning.

The Avoidant, having been injured by enmeshment, commonly creates intensity through risk-taking such as gambling with his life or money, or with compulsive sexuality or work addiction and chemical dependency.

6. The Avoidant Repeats the Cycle by Returning to the Relationship Out of the Fear of Being Left or Guilt, or by Finding a New Partner

Love Avoidants often feel guilty about leaving the relationship. Their role as children with enmeshing parents was to be responsible for that needy person. Caretaking has value to Love Avoidants, so out of guilt they often go back to the Love Addict, who is trying to carry out a plan to get the Love Avoidant back.

When Love Avoidants notice that their partners have given up pursuit and are gone, their fear of abandonment is triggered. They often return to seduce the Love Addict out of fear of abandonment. If Love Avoidants don't return to the same person, they often move on to connect in an addicted way with another partner, often another needy Love Addict.

6.

When Love Addicts Meet Love Avoidants: The Characteristics of Co-Addicted Relationships

Relationships between Love Addicts and Love Avoidants usually involve intensity, obsession, and compulsion, which both parties use to avoid reality and intimacy. The relationships they form constitute a distinctive and separate addictive process, which I call "co-addicted."

THREE CO-ADDICTED RELATIONSHIPS

There are three kinds of co-addicted relationships: between two Love Addicts, between two Love Avoidants, and between a Love Addict and a Love Avoidant.

1. Between Two Love Addicts

A Love Addict and another Love Addict form a very intense relationship. They enmesh with each other, get very dependent on each other, and often exclude other people from the partnership. Many times they even exclude their children, and these children feel very abandoned by the parents' addiction to each other. The intensity, obsession, and compulsion is focused by each partner on the other partner and on the relationship itself.

In some relationships between two Love Addicts, one Love Addict's intense drive toward enmeshment is more forceful than the other's. These forceful attempts to remake the other party to fit his or her fantasy overwhelm this less forceful partner. The less forceful Love Addict, whose similar attempts to remake the forceful partner to fit his or her own fantasy fail, may feel in danger of being engulfed and drained and may therefore shift roles by adopting the characteristics of an Love Avoidant in the relationship.

2. Between Two Love Avoidants

An Love Avoidant and another Love Avoidant form a very low-intensity relationship. They agree to keep intensity low because each of them finds this comfortable; however, they each create intensity, obsession, and compulsion outside the relationship, which quite often does not include the other partner. For example, it could be that one is a work addict in business and the other is intensely involved in church work or another form of volunteer activity. Or perhaps one is an alcoholic and the other a compulsive spender, or compulsive gardener, or compulsively redecorates and remodels their home. Or perhaps one of them avoids the spouse by being a Love Addict when relating to one of the children.

Another possibility is that these two participate together in some form of intensity outside their relationship, thinking they are having a relationship because they are together so much of the time. Actually they use the intensity outside to avoid intimacy within the relationship. For example, a couple can become involved together in compulsive gambling, tournament bridge, square dancing, sailboat racing, and so on. I'm not trying to say that gambling, bridge, dancing, or boat racing are undesirable activities for a couple to share. But such activities may become an obstacle to their relationship when the partners create intensity with these activities to avoid intimacy.

3. Between a Love Addict and a Love Avoidant

A Love Addict and a Love Avoidant form a relationship marked by cycles of positive and negative intensity (which they call love, passion, or romance), until they can't stand it with that partner—and then they leave that person and repeat the cycles with somebody else. Each partner is both attracted and repelled by the other. This paradox is often expressed as, "I can't live with him (or her), but I can't live without him (or her)."

The remainder of this book deals with the co-addicted relationship between a Love Addict and a Love Avoidant, describing in detail how such a relationship operates and what to do about it. Those who find themselves in either of the other two kinds of co-addicted relationships (either Love Addict-Love Addict or Love Avoidant-Love Avoidant) may find helpful guidance here for moving out of these painful places into individual recovery, and from there into a more healthy atmosphere within their relationship. Even one partner getting into recovery can change the old, sick, repetitive patterns and cycles of a co-addicted relationship.

WHAT ADDICTIONS DO FOR A PERSON

An addiction functions in a person's life to remove intolerable reality through a series of obsessive-compulsive experiences. The obsessive-compulsive experience does such a good job of removing the intolerable reality that the person keeps doing it, seeking to feel "comfortable" even though the side effects of the addiction itself become more and more uncomfortable. The addiction becomes a priority in the person's life, becoming more important than anything else and creating harmful consequences, which the addict ignores.

This addictive priority for a Love Addict is the partner and the fantasy the Love Addict has developed about that partner. Love Addicts are obsessed with the partner and seek to create intensity inside the relationship—actually to relate too closely to the point of enmeshment rather than establishing healthy intimacy.

This addictive priority in the Love Avoidant's life is an addiction outside the relationship: alcohol, drugs, sex, work, religion, gambling, spending, being busy. Love Avoidants are interested in creating intensity outside the relationship rather than establishing healthy intimacy within the relationship. Any other addiction will do the job of causing a Love Avoidant to evade intimacy within the relationship by focusing on the outside addiction.

As we have seen, a co-addicted relationship is often a romantic-sexual relationship between a woman (the Love Addict) and a man (the Love Avoidant), although sometimes the reverse is true. And as we have seen, not all co-addicted relationships are romantic-sexual. Almost any kind of relationship between two human beings can become co-addicted.

BOTH ROLES CAN BE EXPERIENCED BY ONE PERSON

To make matters more complex, it is possible for one person to exhibit the traits of both roles. A person who is a Love Avoidant in a primary relationship, for instance, can become a Love Addict outside the relationship. For example, let's say Marty is a sex addict, married to Sharon, a Love Addict. Marty is the Love Avoidant within the marriage. But outside this primary relationship, as a sex addict Marty may have an affair with Jackie, who is another sex addict. While Marty is avoiding intimacy with Sharon in his marriage, he may act as a Love Addict when relating to Jackie. (Yes, read that again, slowly.) The possibilities are endless and sometimes quite intricate.

As codependents, both parties experience an inner failure of the relationship with themselves. But their behavior in the co-addicted relationship reflects this inner failure in different ways. As we've seen, the core of a healthy relationship is the exchange of intimacy at one or more of four levels: physical, sexual, emotional, and intellectual.

In healthy intimate relationships, internal boundaries[1] protect us and keep us comfortable when we receive input from someone—a compliment, a grievance, an expression of feeling, or just an acknowledgment of a difficulty within the relationship. Internal boundaries also keep us from being abusive when we give input to someone else. Good internal boundaries allow us to be serene while we risk sharing our reality. Without good boundaries there is much to fear about being intimate.

---

2 Boundaries are more fully described in *Facing Codependence,* by Pia Mellody, with Andrea Wells Miller and J. Keith Miller (San Francisco: Harper & Row, 1989), and in a two-tape lecture by Pia Mellody entitled "Boundaries," which can be ordered from Featuka Enterprises, Inc., 651 Chaparral Road, Wickenburg, AZ 85390. Phone and fax: 520-684-7484; 1-800-626-6779.

What is exchanged between two addict-codependents is very different from the exchange of intimacy in a healthy relationship. Codependents lack healthy boundaries (a core symptom of codependence). Without adequate internal boundaries, neither partner can be intimate—that is, neither can experience this exchange without either trying to fix or change the other partner, or defensively justifying themselves and arguing about the other person's reality, or abusing the partner with so-called "honesty," or with sarcasm, exaggeration, ridicule, name-calling, or other violations of internal boundaries.

INTERACTION BETWEEN THE TWO

It could be said that the Love Addict is kind of a liberal about relationships and the Love Avoidant is kind of a conservative. Love Addicts are constantly seeking change to improve things in the relationship and to get what they want—more contact, more care. On the other hand, Love Avoidants want acceptance of the status quo, and so they work to keep the relationship stable, predictable, and unemotional; Love Avoidants don't see change as an advantage. Love Addicts think that Love Avoidants are the problem because they won't change. But when the Love Avoidant contemplates a change requested by the Love Addict, the Love Avoidant thinks that to change is to capitulate to or be controlled by somebody else. Stalemate.

The Love Avoidant avoids intimacy and is hypersensitive to any sense of being controlled. The Love Addict seeks enmeshment and is hypersensitive to any sense of being left.

WHY LOVE ADDICTS AND LOVE AVOIDANTS ARE ATTRACTED TO EACH OTHER

With all this conflict, it may seem strange that these people could ever have been attracted to each other. But it is important to note that each person is first attracted to the other specifically because of the "familiar" traits that the other exhibits. These traits, although painful, are familiar from childhood abuse experiences. Neither a Love Addict nor a Love Avoidant is usually attracted to a non-addicted person. When either encounters such a person, the response is something like "Gosh, he's boring," or "I don't think we have enough in common," or "The chemistry isn't there for me," or "She's too independent for me to relate to." And it's true: The elements that keep the familiar but devastating process of a co-addicted relationship alive are not present in a relationship with a non-addicted person. Until the Love Addict and Love Avoidant acquire more healthy ways of thinking, feeling, and behaving in a relationship, healthy people will continue to appear less attractive. Just changing partners to a healthier person without doing the work of recovery will not solve the problem.

But why specifically are these two addict-codependents attracted to one another? What are the traits that attract them? I believe several factors are involved.

What Attracts Love Addicts to Love Avoidants

At least three factors are involved in the attraction a Love Addict feels toward a Love Avoidant: (1) attraction to what is familiar; (2) attraction to situations in which there is hope that childhood wounds can be healed; and (3) attraction to the possibility for fulfillment of the fantasy created in childhood.

1. ATTRACTION TO WHAT IS FAMILIAR

In our family of origin, we are taught how to be intimate our family's way. How our caregivers operate in their relationship becomes very familiar to us as children. As dysfunctional as the relationship may be, we as children become accustomed to it, and in many ways that familiarity feels comfortable or safe. When we grow up and look for our own partner, on some level we are attracted to people who remind us of the people who raised us.

Because the sense of abandonment and disconnectedness that Love Addicts experience in their family of origin teaches them as children to be quiet, alone, needless, and wantless—so as not to bother the parents—they are later unconsciously attracted to people who don't try to attach to them very much.

The people who attract them are usually involved in many things, often one or more addictions. Such people appear to really take care of themselves because they're so busy and intense. Love Addicts are familiar with people who are involved in many activities and don't have time to give them much attention.

2. ATTRACTION TO SITUATIONS IN WHICH EARLY CHILDHOOD WOUNDS CAN BE RESOLVED

A part of self-esteem was wounded in Love Addicts' childhoods, since abandonment sent the message that they were not worth being with. A large part of their magnetic pull toward Love Avoidants is that Love Addicts find people who are walking away from them very attractive. They may attempt to heal the wound to their self-esteem by trying to resolve the issue they were never powerful enough to solve as children: making an abandoning person connect with them, thereby restoring their own sense of preciousness and getting the parenting they didn't get as children.

I deeply wanted my father to be there with me. I wanted his attention as evidence of his love, but he did not come through for me. I think that by being attracted to people who weren't there for me and trying to find a way to get these people to give me the time and attention I didn't get as a child, I was trying to work out that old issue about my relationship to my father. Such behavior is more than just meeting a need for attention; it's an attempt to heal the old wound that we received in childhood.

3. ATTRACTION TO POTENTIAL FULFILLMENT OF CHILDHOOD FANTASY

Love Addicts also look for someone to fulfill their childhood fantasy of a rescuer who will protect and comfort them, a person to become their Higher Power. Healthy people who expect them to have opinions, who don't volunteer to solve their problems, who don't ooze with "seduction," and who don't engage in intense arguments are not interesting to Love Addicts. They may think of such people as boring, insensitive, or strange. On the other hand, a Love Avoidant's take-control manner, seductive charms, and intense control of arguments is electrifying.

What Attracts Love Avoidants to Love Addicts

At least two of the factors described above are involved in the attraction of the Love Avoidant for the Love Addict: (1) attraction to what is familiar, and (2) attraction to situations in which there is the possibility of healing the wounds of childhood.

1. ATTRACTION TO WHAT IS FAMILIAR

Love Avoidants are accustomed to needy, dependent, helpless people whom they can rescue, which gives them control and a feeling of safety and power. Their emotional radar scans for someone to rescue; and when they pick up the right signal, Love Avoidants move in very seductively and powerfully. People who think for themselves, say directly what they mean, solve their own problems, don't get caught up in intense fighting, and take care of themselves reasonably well are not interesting to Love Avoidants. In fact, they might be considered too independent, too smart for their own good, or—in the case of an independent woman—not feminine enough.

2. ATTRACTION TO SITUATIONS IN WHICH OLD CHILDHOOD WOUNDS CAN BE RESOLVED

The childhood wounds of the Love Avoidant come from being drained, used, and abandoned. Love Avoidants are frequently attracted to those who do not have power, are dependent and vulnerable, and seem easy to control. Love Avoidants believe that relationships with such people will heal the wounds of their childhood enmeshment by protecting them from being engulfed or drained.

What Alienates Love Addicts and Love Avoidants

At the same time Love Addicts and Love Avoidants are attracted to one another, they are also eventually repelled by each other. Love Addicts get abandoned when Love Avoidants start up their addiction. The Love Addict's pain, fear, and anger are coupled with old childhood feelings from the original abandonment experience, producing intense discomfort.

Love Avoidants begin to feel controlled and engulfed by the neediness of the Love Addict, coupled with the draining pressure put on them to be the caretaker, to be there for the Love Addict, and to solve all difficulties. So they are attracted by the familiarity but repelled by the repetitive abuse they experience.

We have seen that both partners in a co-addicted relationship have the same two fears of abandonment and intimacy. Figure 3 illustrates how the *conscious* fear of one partner is the *unconscious* fear of the other.

	Conscious Fear	Unconscious Fear
Love Addict	Abandonment	Intimacy
Love Avoidant	Intimacy (Engulfment)	Abandonment

Figure 3

In the course of the relationship, the distancing maneuvers of the Love Avoidant to escape the intensity of the Love Addict's pursuit trigger the abandonment fears of the Love Addict. The Love Addict winds up abandoned because the Love Avoidant can't stand the neediness and the intensity that the Love Addict keeps creating within the relationship.

In turn, the Love Addict's extreme neediness and intense pursuit of the partner triggers the engulfment fears of the Love Avoidant; and the Love Avoidant winds up getting engulfed by the neediness and persistence of the Love Addict. Each of them experiences their primary conscious fear, and their own behavior actually provokes a great deal of the behavior in the other that they find intolerable.

The Co-Addicted Tango
The Love Addict eventually becomes exhausted with the pursuit, gives up, and turns away to begin either getting well or moving into another relationship or an addiction to cover the pain. After a while the Love Avoidant partner notices that he or she is no longer being pursued. This triggers deep, underlying abandonment fears, and the Love Avoidant turns around to try to get close to the Love Addict again. One is running and the other one is chasing almost all the time. When the one who is chasing finally gets close to the one running away, they both erupt into intensity, either a brief romantic interlude or a terrific fight.

The Love Avoidant usually becomes seductive as a way of reconnecting, and starts doing all the things that the partner always wanted him or her to do. The Love Addict says, "Oh, wow," turns around to face the partner, exclaiming in joy, "Oh, you love me," and goes toward the Love Avoidant. When the Love Avoidant sees the Love Addict coming, with all that neediness and intensity, he or she pulls away and runs, reversing the direction of the dance once again. Their tango produces what I call positive and negative intensity.

Positive and Negative Intensity

As we can see, while there may be variations from couple to couple, co-addicted relationships have a fairly predictable pattern. Figure 4 shows each of the wheels we have already examined in previous chapters. Now we will trace how the behavior of each partner triggers the reaction of the other, and how that reaction then triggers the original partner into a reaction.

The left wheel represents the Love Addict's emotional cycle; imagine that it rotates counterclockwise. The right wheel represents the cycle of the Love Avoidant; imagine that it rotates clockwise. Notice that now there are cogs on each wheel, like the cogs in the gears of a machine. The cogs on each wheel mesh with those on the other wheel, driving both wheels around the cycles. Each participant in the relationship experiences his or her own individual cycle, but the interaction between the two of them creates the co-addicted relationship experience, an intense, chaotic, jolting encounter.

THE LOVE ADDICT'S CYCLE OF
POSITIVE AND NEGATIVE INTENSITY

A Love Addict who feels the seductive pursuit of the Love Avoidant experiences positive intensity. The Love Addict, turning toward the Love Avoidant, continues to experience an emotional "high," or positive intensity, because that childhood fantasy is trig-

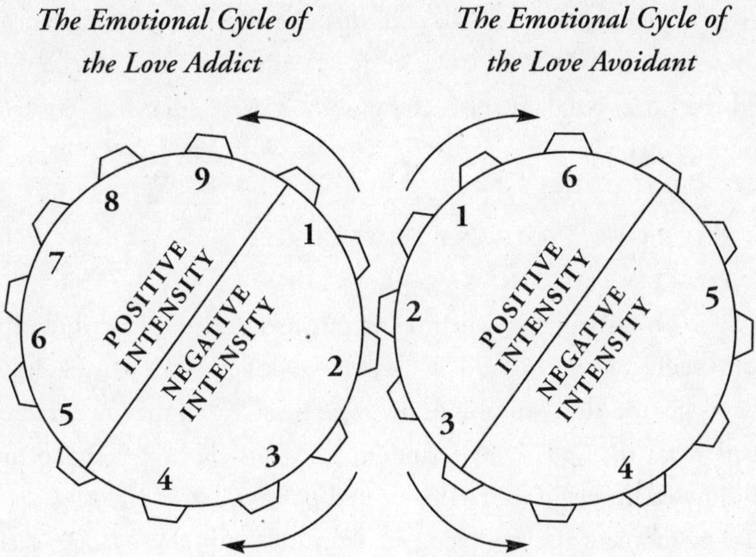

The Emotional Cycle of the Love Addict

The Emotional Cycle of the Love Avoidant

THE LOVE ADDICT

1. is *attracted* to the seductiveness and apparant "power" of the Love Avoidant.

2. feels *high* as the fantasy is triggered.

3. feels *relief* from pain of loneliness, emptiness, and not mattering to partner.

4. shows more neediness and *denies reality* of the Avoidant's walls.

5. develops awareness of partner's walls and behavior outside the relationship and *denial crumbles.*

6. enters *withdrawl.*

7. *obsesses* about how to get the Love Avoidant to return or how to get even.

8. *compulsively acts out* obsessive plans.

9. *repeats the cycle* with the Love Avoidant, if he or she returns, or with a new partner.

THE LOVE AVOIDANT

1. is unable to say no to the relationship.

2. connects to the Love Addict with *seduction.*

3. feels *engulfed* anyway, moves to a wall of anger or resentment and gets critical of partner.

4. uses resentment or sense of being a victim to move to a wall of distance.

5. seeks intensity outside the relationship in order to feel "alive" and have a life of his or her own.

6. *repeats the cycle* by returning to the relationship out of fear of being left or guilt, or by finding a new relationship.

Figure 4. How Each Emotional Cycle Drives the Other

gered. When the partner bolts and runs, these feelings change to negative intensity. When the Love Addict finally turns away once more and the Love Avoidant starts chasing, the Love Addict feels positive intensity again.

THE LOVE AVOIDANT'S CYCLE OF
POSITIVE AND NEGATIVE INTENSITY

The Love Avoidant, when being pursued, feels positive intensity from being in control and in power—as long as the Love Addict doesn't get too close with his or her neediness. When the Love Addict turns away, the underlying abandonment fears are triggered and the Love Avoidant begins to feel panic and pain, negative intensity.

The moment the one being chased turns and they're facing each other, they're each experiencing positive intensity at the same time. But as the relationship continues, that time of mutual positive intensity gets shorter and shorter until it's reduced to a split second before they're back into fighting again and creating negative intensity.

Our Culture Considers This
Behavior "True Love"

Although much of our society calls all this "normal" in a love relationship, this swing from positive to negative intensity has little to do with love. I believe that our cultural ways of looking at passion and love are dysfunctional. What we call passion and love is really intensity; and we call it "normal," meaning that many relationships are like this. But while this sort of addictive process may be common, in my opinion it isn't healthy. In a codependent-addictive relationship, one or both parties are almost always in delusion about the fact that their relationship is based not on love but on a form of positive and negative intensity that they mistake for passion and love.

Who's the Victim Here?

The combined immaturity of each partner makes a co-addicted relationship intense, chaotic, and undependable. Both parties are equally responsible for creating this intensity and chaos. Neither one is necessarily any healthier or more offensive than the other. In their own ways, each abuses the other. The Love Addict may look like the helpless victim and the Love Avoidant may look insensitive or mean, but both offend each other in major ways; neither is the sole victim.

What complicates matters is that in a "love" relationship we expect our partners to behave with maturity even though we ourselves may be deluded about our own maturity and are acting like whining, spoiled brats or raging offenders. I'll never forget that day I broke through the denial and delusion about my immaturity and began to see the reality of the person with whom my partner was living—me. Coming out of denial was quite a shock, but I believe it was the beginning of my recovery.

The cycles we have been discussing are immature, fruitless, and pain-filled. Fortunately there is a way of relating that is healthier and more fulfilling than this.

A Brief Look At
Healthy Relationships

Many of us think that the right partner will complete a missing part of ourselves, finally making us feel whole. We also believe that this ideal lover will reveal the meaning of life to us. But each one of us has the potential to feel whole and fulfilled from within ourselves to the extent that we can develop our competence in self-love, self-protection, self-awareness, self-care, and self-containment.

In addition, each one of us searches for and eventually finds the meaning of life for ourselves, rather than looking to our partner to reveal it to us. The only meaning our partner can reveal is the meaning of his or her life. Our lives are ours; our partner's life is his or hers. No one can give us the ultimate answers for our own lives. We discover our own meaning because it is relevant to us. Trying to force ourselves to fit into another person's concept of the meaning of life won't work, because that concept probably doesn't fit us. Likewise, trying to make someone else fit into our concept of the meaning of life won't work either, because that concept probably won't fit the other person.

To me a healthy relationship is not based on obsession and compulsion; it does not thrive on positive and negative intensity. I believe that in healthy relationships, as Dr. Jordan Paul and Margaret Paul have written, you are able to nurture others in a way that promotes their emotional and spiritual growth and promotes their taking responsibility for themselves, thereby increasing their self-esteem.[2]

When you love yourself, you are able to nurture yourself, focus on your own emotional and spiritual growth, and take responsibility for yourself, thereby increasing your own sense of self-esteem. When one partner is asked for acts of intimacy or support by the other, each person can say yes or no in a healthy way, without either partner being diminished. The self-esteem of each individual blossoms when nurtured within a healthy relationship.

A MEANS OF RECOVERY

As I have learned by experience and by observation more about this painful process of the co-addictive relationship, I have found

2See Dr. Jordan Paul and Margaret Paul, *From Conflict to Caring* (Minneapolis, MN: Compcare, 1988).

some helpful and effective tools for stopping the addictive process and entering recovery. In the rest of this book, we will explore them together. We will also look at some marks of a healthy relationship, so that when you have enough recovery from Love Addiction, or any other addictions that have damaged your relationships, you can begin to set some realistic goals for yourself in future relationships.

Part II

THE
RECOVERY PROCESS

7

What to Do About Your Co-Addicted Relationship

Through my own struggles and those of many people I have counseled, I have learned that there is a recovery process for co-addicted relationships that gets results. It is optimal if both people are involved in the process; but if one person will not try these recovery methods, the other can still benefit greatly from them. That person will, I believe, find a greater level of comfort either within the same relationship or without it. This is especially true for the Love Addict.

RECOVERY IS NOTICEABLE TO OTHERS

For a while I went through my own cycles of love addiction while giving seminars about it. That was a very difficult experience for me, but I kept on working through this recovery process. One evening when I was speaking, a woman in the audience whom I know said to me, "You really look a lot better, Pia!" And because of her comment I became aware that after I managed to stop going around the emotional cycle and got through withdrawal, my life did get much better. I can personally declare that there is hope.

While it is only fair to warn you that going through the recovery process is a difficult and rather miserable experience, I also believe most people who are sick of living this self-defeating way can do what it takes to recover. We experience difficulty and misery while stuck in the cycles, or we try to avoid this difficulty and misery by avoiding relationships altogether, only to find a different kind of pain from being alone. The pain we experience during recovery is more manageable because it is accompanied by hope, since we are now headed for improvement. We decide to face ourselves and enter a process that offers eventually to heal the pain as we confront the addiction and our denial about it and step consciously into recovery. As many have heard me say often, "Hug your demons or they'll bite you in the ass."

THE PHASES OF RECOVERY

How do we get out of the addictive, driven quality in a relationship and into a more healthy way of relating? I believe we need to work through the following four steps, which we will explore throughout the rest of Part II.

1. Begin addressing any apparent addictive processes outside the co-addicted relationship (alcoholism, eating disorders, and so on).
2. Disengage from the addictive part of the relationship process. (More about how to do this follows.)
3. Enter therapy, if necessary, for help releasing your old stored-up feelings from childhood abuse experiences. A few people can come to terms with old childhood feelings of abandonment or enmeshment on their own. But in my expe-

rience, most people who recover from toxic relationships as adults first need therapeutic help with their internal residue of unresolved and harmful feelings from childhood.

4. Work on underlying symptoms of codependence.

After undertaking these steps, most people are ready to reenter a relationship. If you have temporarily disengaged from your current relationship in order to get into recovery (without actually having ended the relationship), you will probably be ready to reenter that relationship when you have dealt with the four phases of recovery listed above. On the other hand, you may be almost forced into recovery because your partner has left for good, or because events have transpired that lead to the final ending of the relationship. To give yourself the best opportunity to enjoy a more healthy way of relating, I suggest staying out of new relationships until you have moved through the four steps outlined above.

If your former relationship terminates permanently and no new relationship comes along for a while (or at all), it is a sure sign of recovery if you are able to resist the attraction to a rescuing Love Avoidant or to a helpless, needy Love Addict who invites rescuing (whichever role you've played). At times the choice may be to be to go without a relationship rather than go through a co-addicted experience again. If this choice to remain without a relationship is a conscious choice stemming from your recovery as opposed to a way to avoid facing the problem, I see it as healthy. But the healthy choice does call for finding creative ways to meet your need for appropriate physical and emotional nurture and intimacy. We will look at that process, and I will describe some ways you can try to look for a person with whom you may be able to begin a more healthy relationship.

Another encouraging factor is that as you get healthier in your codependence recovery, you may become attracted to healthier people and find that healthier people are attracted to you. The healthier the person to whom you are attracted, the more likely the person will be able to give you warm, personal regard regularly.

ARRESTING ALL ADDICTIONS

At least three and possibly four addiction processes occur in a co-addicted relationship:

1. The love addiction of the Love Addict;
2. The addiction(s) of the Love Avoidant;
3. The co-addicted relationship itself; and
4. The other addictions possibly used at times by the Love Addict to medicate the pain of love addiction.

We have already defined the co-addicted relationship as a toxic exchange of positive and negative intensity between the two addicts who are codependent; an experience that the participants can't leave but can't tolerate either. In this sense it is very much like an addiction process.

Arresting an addiction is simple to explain, although not always easy to do. The way to arrest each of these categories of addictions is the same: (1) Confront the addiction by acknowledging that the symptoms are operating in your life; (2) examine the harmful consequences created by the addiction issues; (3) intervene on the addictive cycle; and (4) experience withdrawal.

1. Confront the Addiction Within Yourself

The experience of recognizing oneself as an addict is not very pleasant, because along with that acknowledgment comes the emotional pain of loss. The results created by the addiction may seem to be gratifying: emotional highs, lots of excitement and intensity, and medication of intolerable reality. Love addiction specifically brings connection to someone, painful as it is, and it works well for a while. Without whatever addictions you are now confronting, you will need to learn to face reality as it is and deal with it.

LOVE ADDICTION AND THE
CO-ADDICTED RELATIONSHIP

It is a commonly held rule among many counselors who treat addicts that no one can recover from an addiction without recognizing it as an addictive process. As long as Love Addicts don't see both their own patterns of relating and the relationship process itself as addictions, I believe they are almost impossible to treat. If you are in denial that you are an addict, there is virtually nothing anybody can do to help you until you move into reality—the reality that you are an addict. This almost always means waiting until the pain is so severe that it cracks the shell of the denial.

SECONDARY ADDICTIONS

At a certain point in their cycle, Love Addicts encounter times when the pain is immense, and may use some other addiction (such as sex addiction, alcoholism, drug addiction, addictive television viewing, work addiction, religious addiction, an eating disorder) to relieve the pain. They often have to arrest not only love addiction, but also any other addictions they have used to mask the painful reality of the love addiction.

ADDICTIONS OF THE LOVE AVOIDANT

Love Avoidants also need to confront any addictions before they can deal successfully with the co-addicted relationship. Love Avoidants usually find it extremely difficult (if not impossible) to get out of the co-addicted relationship process unless they break away from their outside addiction(s) first.

It is very difficult for a practicing addict to be in a mature and healthy relationship. Addicts create only dysfunctional relationships.

An addict may stumble into a relationship with a non-addicted person while on the rebound from a relationship with a Love Addict, but will most likely develop a dysfunctional relationship even if the other party is not a Love Addict or another Love Avoidant. In my opinion the best hope a person has of experiencing a healthy relationship with someone is to enter recovery from any addictive processes and from symptoms of codependence, then use discretion in selecting a non-addicted partner.

Whether we are Love Addicts or Love Avoidants, we need to face all of our addictions.

In my opinion the underpinnings of any addiction (other than alcohol or drug addiction) have to do with untreated codependence, the inability to deal with our reality, which leads us to medicate the pain of it with one or more addictions. I also have come to believe that Love Addiction usually cannot be treated or possibly even recognized until the addict-codependent has sufficient recovery from the codependence to be able to face life with more internal comfort; for it is the healing of the core symptoms of codependence that brings this internal comfort.

I also believe that on some level Love Addicts are aware that they are too immature to take care of themselves and must cling to somebody. When Love Addicts experience recovery in the first four symptoms of codependence, they have the tools to confront Love Addiction. Codependence recovery, especially in the area of self-care and self-nurture, gives Love Addicts enough stability to stand the withdrawal from the love addiction when they finally recognize it and become willing to go into withdrawal.

So Love Addicts must often begin by arresting any other addictions that are going on, experiencing withdrawal from them, and beginning codependence recovery before they can go on to the more difficult process of facing the love addiction and entering withdrawal from it.

2. Examine the Harmful Consequences of the Addiction

When we examine the harmful consequences of each addiction, we can begin to experience the pain that motivates us to stop the addiction, endure withdrawal, and learn healthy responses to our painful reality, thereby reducing or eliminating the harmful consequences of our addictions.

3. Intervene on the Addictive Cycle

In situations in which you have been engaged in your addictive process, you need to stop and be willing to go into withdrawal and stay there without returning to the addictive experience, until the withdrawal has passed. For example, you need to stop chasing somebody who doesn't want to be with you; stop having sex with inappropriate people; stop drinking; stop overeating; stop overworking. You need to stop whatever is the focus of your addictive behavior.

4. Experience Withdrawal

When an addicted person stops using a substance or behavior to which he or she is addicted, that person enters withdrawal, an indicator that the person was truly addicted to whatever has been taken away. Withdrawal is a series of uncomfortable symptoms that people experience when the addictive substance is removed. The withdrawal experience can be confirmed if the withdrawal symptoms disappear when the substance is reinstituted. For example, if you are addicted to sugar and you stop eating sugar, the headaches caused by withdrawal can be severe. But if you then eat some chocolate candy or ice cream, and the pain leaves, you can be pretty sure you were in withdrawal from an addiction.

The withdrawal symptoms are, therefore, what drive us back to the substance or behavior to which we are addicted. The symptoms may be physical, intellectual, emotional, or spiritual in nature. In the case of love addiction they are mainly emotional, whereas in alcoholism the withdrawal symptoms are often more physical in nature, as well as emotional.

To make it through this painful period, we need a consistent outside source of help and encouragement. This can be found in Twelve-Step meetings. Love Addicts or sex addicts can go to Sex and Love Addicts Anonymous (SLAA). Al-Anon, a Twelve-Step group for the friends and relatives of alcoholics, can also provide support for the withdrawal pains of love addiction. The men and women who love alcoholics are often Love Addicts who can support each other in detaching from an Love Avoidant partner who abandons their relationship through drinking. Alcoholics go to Alcoholics Anonymous (AA). Drug addicts go to NarcAnon (NA) or AA. Compulsive overeaters, bulimics, anorexics, and food addicts go to Overeaters Anonymous (OA). Recovering people go to whatever addiction meeting we need that will give us the support to stay in withdrawal.

Another form of support we may need is therapy. Those who seek help from a counselor need to choose an addiction specialist who knows about withdrawal from alcoholism, drug addiction, overwork, food addiction, sex addiction, and love addiction.

Sometimes some of us need medical attention. Severe alcoholics or drug addicts need medication to keep from dying from the effects of withdrawal. People who are in the throes of love addiction withdrawal (described in chapter 9) also may need medication for their withdrawal symptoms. Love addiction withdrawal is not a simple experience, because the intense emotional pain and depression is often experienced as a desire to harm oneself and can sometimes lead to suicide or homicide, or homicide followed by suicide. Newspapers report daily deaths from this addiction. In my opinion, some of these people need to be supported with antidepressant medication.

Treating an addiction involves owning the addiction, facing the harmful consequences, stopping the addictive behavior, going into withdrawal, and treating the withdrawal. Once you are sober or stable after the effects of withdrawal from your addictions, you are ready to move into the next phase of recovery.

8.

PUTTING THE
RELATIONSHIP ON HOLD

Marriage counseling can often help couples who wish to improve their relationship. But when the marriage exhibits the characteristics of a co-addicted relationship, I believe traditional counseling needs to wait until each partner has begun recovery from other addictions and from codependence.

One of the main problems in co-addicted relationships is that because of their untreated codependence, neither partner is mature enough to have a healthy relationship. Self-esteem problems and difficulty setting boundaries make it very difficult for each partner to cope with negative feedback from the other, or with doing insight work with a counselor in the presence of the partner. Such vital work is overwhelming enough to do in private; often it is much too threatening to allow one's partner to watch. In such cases each partner needs to detach from the other with regard to recovery issues, and proceed with his or her own addiction and codependence recovery separately.

Some relationships, however, have not deteriorated to such toxic levels by the time the partners decide to do something about the relationship. If each partner has some degree of maturity and addiction recovery, the couple may be able to enter marriage counseling and do pretty well, realizing that they each need to do separate codependence recovery also.

The procedure I'm about to describe for putting a relationship on hold is for relationships that are so toxic that the partners can't say things like "When you do so-and-so, I feel angry" without a lot of explosion or chaos. All relationships are not so toxic that the parties must detach in this way while they do their own recovery. But so many are this toxic that I want to say clearly that such detachment (within the bonds of the relationship, if possible) may be necessary, and in any case this detachment is extremely helpful for getting into recovery more effectively.

Later, after doing some separate codependence recovery, the partners can begin to work on issues together. For instance, if the partners can begin to say, "When you did this, I felt this way," they are beginning to work together to practice sharing emotional intimacy with each other; they are working on the third core symptom of codependence, owning one's reality and sharing it appropriately.

How Long Is a Reasonable Recovery Period?

I have found that the total recovery time for detoxification from addiction and childhood trauma experience, followed by a period of codependence recovery and relationship recovery, is usually three to five years. That doesn't mean you have to have your relationship on hold for three to five years. After a period of up to about six months of having the relationship on hold to get started on your own recovery, it might take an additional three to six months to reenter the relationship and develop reasonable comfort within it after one has begun serious work on the major addictions and the core symptoms of codependence. This varies from partnership to partnership. The rest of the three to five years involves each person continuing to do recovery work on the symptoms of codependence. During this recovery period many important aspects of the marriage can continue, even though the parties are not working on their addictive-codependent issues together.

DISENGAGING FROM THE ADDICTIVE PROCESS OF YOUR CURRENT RELATIONSHIP

During the period in which you are confronting any addictions and entering codependence recovery, it is usually best to do very little with regard to fixing the relationship. I recommend disengaging from it until you have experienced addiction recovery and a certain amount of codependence recovery.

In some cases, however, the Love Addict partner does not have the ability to take care of his or her own needs and wants and so cannot tolerate withdrawal from, or even within, the relationship. In such cases couples may need to wait until that symptom has improved.

Even though the Love Avoidant partner was not for the most part present in the relationship because of other addictions, the times he or she was present in the relationship were usually episodes of extreme intensity—either grand passion or fighting and violence (verbal, physical, whatever) or both. The Love Avoidant needs to disengage from these addictive parts of the relationship—the extreme intensity of it. Although this may seem like more abandonment, it is a necessary and temporary phase of recovery that gives the Love Addict time to heal enough to be able to maintain a healthy relationship later on.

The procedure for arresting the addictive process of the relationship is the same as for any other addiction already dealt with: Face the fact that it is an addiction, own the harmful consequences, then intervene on the addictive cycle and enter withdrawal.

Many individuals may find it necessary to go to a counselor while attempting to put the relationship on hold. I have found that many Love Addicts who enter the withdrawal phase from a co-addicted relationship usually can't do it effectively on their own (although it can be done by some).

HOW TO PUT THE RELATIONSHIP ON HOLD

Putting a relationship on hold doesn't necessarily mean separating or getting a divorce, although some couples do need a physical separation. It also doesn't mean that the partners have no contact. It just means that the partners eliminate any contact that leads to fighting, intensity, and painful feelings, or trying to deal with the issues of the co-addicted relationship with each other. Emotional interactions, criticism, and major problem-solving are kept to a minimum or eliminated, if possible. Any problems that can't be avoided (such as whether to send your son to private school or how to finance braces for your daughter) need to be approached with a third party who can moderate, such as a counselor.

HOW MUCH INTIMATE CONTACT MUST BE AVOIDED VARIES FROM COUPLE TO COUPLE

Intimacy (sharing and receiving reality from another person) requires having enough boundaries to know who you are and who the other person is. With boundaries you can keep yourself comfortable while you listen to someone give you his or her reality. Intimacy also includes having the ability to say no to your partner without becoming an offender. Intimacy can be physical, sexual, emotional, and intellectual.

Some partners can share and receive reality in one or more of those four areas without offending the other, while in other areas they can't. For instance, some couples can be sexual but cannot try to settle differences about emotional needs. Some couples can't relate in any of the areas without getting into fights and painful feelings. Once a couple realizes that there are parts of intimacy they can't share, they can ask a counselor to help them negotiate what kind of intimacy can continue and what has to stop in order to intervene on the addictive part of the relationship process. The counselor can help the couple clarify the problem areas that need to be negotiated, and set up a regular meeting time so that the couple can do this part of the intimate contact with the counselor as a guide.

CLOSING DOWN THE RELATIONSHIP

Detachment from the addictive parts of the relationship means not trying to do any kind of intense relating with your partner. Treat each other in a very pleasant way and go on about your own business. Keep just enough interaction in the "allowed" areas to feel some partnership, but don't interact about anything in the areas of intimacy you know are off limits. If all four areas are off limits, just stay on a polite superficial level, using good manners and detachment.

If your partner flings out an opening for hostility, do not respond directly, not even to say, "We're not supposed to deal with things like that." Just continue to be pleasant, but close your mouth and breathe; sit on your hands if necessary, but don't discuss anything that's irritating.

I've found that following these rules effectively allows each partner to detach from the relationship.

1. Practice "the three gets" from Al-Anon: Get off your partner's back, get out of your partner's way, and get on with your life.
2. Do not "bomb" your partner with anger or seduction (this process will be explained later).
3. Notice what is happening to your partner so you can see who your partner is.
4. Notice what is going on with you.
5. Do not respond to any bombs of anger or seduction from your partner. That doesn't mean never to have sex, but to avoid manipulative, seductive, controlling sex, or fighting and anger.

THE THREE GETS OF AL-ANON

To get off your partner's back means to stop looking intently at the other party, to stop paying attention to what your partner is doing or not doing, and regard it as none of your business. It is helpful merely to *notice* what your partner is doing or not doing; this can help break through the fantasy you have created about who the person is in order to see who he or she *really* is. To get off your partner's back means to cease *responding* to what your partner is doing or not doing by expressing an opinion or feeling to him or her, offering a "suggestion" or solution, asking your partner to change, and so on. If you have difficulty stopping such responding, then I recommend that for now you avoid even noticing and observing your partner as much as possible.

To get out of your partner's way means to try not to interfere with or even observe and evaluate what's going on in your partner's life.

Getting out of the way of the other person means to try not to give helpful advice or negative comments, not to help the other person avoid catastrophe, but also not to create a catastrophe. Make all of your partner's observed behavior none of your business.

To get on with your life means to get into recovery from any addictions you have and from codependence. Most of all, for Love Addicts getting on with your life means to learn how to take care of your needs and wants yourself, to take adult responsibility for your own care, and to stop trying to get somebody else to do it for you. Also learn to focus on how to value yourself, how to set your boundaries, and how to own your reality.

BOMBING TO RECONNECT WITH THE PARTNER

When you have effectively accomplished this detachment, the intensity subsides and the environment may get extremely quiet, especially in comparison to the way it was. When the intensity is gone, it may seem as if you have nothing left in the relationship, because intensity was practically all you had in the first place.

When the relationship gets this quiet, each partner becomes uncomfortable because each is accustomed to the ebb and flow of toxic intensity. Also, the discomfort of the quietness is emphasized by the fact that neither partner knows how to be intimate in a healthy way. Love Addicts are usually the first to become uncomfortable, because they are not engaged in any compulsive behavior to get the Love Avoidant to "love" them. Love Avoidants feel uncomfortable later, when the fear of abandonment starts to surface. When either one feels the discomfort of detachment, they are tempted to do something I call "bombing" to create the old, familiar intensity with the partner, which feels intimate even if it doesn't feel good. Bombing attempts to create so much intensity, either with angry fights or with forms of seduction, that the partner will break the detachment, respond, and reconnect, even if the connection is toxic.

A Word to the Love Addict

When calm and quiet descend on the relationship, your abandonment issues are almost immediately triggered. Right away, you may have a compelling urge to fire off some intensity bombs to get reconnected to your partner. Here are two ways you as a Love Addict might bomb your partner. An "anger bomb" is picking a fight and being angry so that you can get the Love Avoidant to emotionally connect with you, because it's less fearful to be fighting than to be silent. Another way to bomb is with a "seduction bomb." There are two kinds of "seduction bombs." One involves displaying helplessness, and the other is being sexually provocative.

As a Love Addict seeking to disengage from your relationship, you need to resist such bombing. You must work at tolerating the silence. Mature relationships can have long episodes of silence in them. They are not based on creating intensity but on having safety and serenity. By going to Twelve-Step meetings and talking to a sponsor, you can participate in authentic intimacy and begin to discover alternatives to bombing.

Although at first the quietness in the relationship gives relief to the Love Avoidant, eventually his or her own abandonment issues are triggered and he or she will then want to bomb also. You, the Love Addict, need to be prepared not to respond if this happens. The best way I know to avoid responding is the same method of avoiding either kind of bomb. Close your mouth and breathe, observing your partner and noting how he or she is attempting with anger or seduction to connect with you.

A Word to the Love Avoidant

Disengaging through a conscious decision to enter recovery rather than through outside addictions usually gives you, the Love Avoidant, a sense of relief and happiness at first, but some painful withdrawal symptoms often set in a little later.

In the meantime, however, if your Love Addict partner is not on a recovery path, your disengagement from the intensity of the relationship could very well lead your partner to try to escalate the intensity because of fear of abandonment. Even a Love Addict attempting to get into recovery may find it difficult to avoid such attempts at emotional connection at first. If the Love Addict should attempt any bombing, you need to avoid responding and escalating the intensity. The best way I know to do that is just to close your mouth and breathe. You must work at resisting the temptation to respond to bombs, keeping the detachment and the quietness in the relationship. Continually remind yourself that mature relationships can have long episodes of silence in them.

Eventually your own abandonment issues or guilt may be triggered, and you too will want to bomb. Anger bombs may be tempting, as may seduction bombs, which include either being sexually seductive or offering to rescue your partner from some inconvenience or difficulty. By this time your partner may have calmed down and learned how to keep from bombing you, so the roles are reversed for a time. The formerly clutching Love Addict may seem more like an Love Avoidant in comparison to former behavior.

METHODS OF BOMBING

Before this detachment process begins, it's very helpful for each partner to list all the ways you can think of that you bomb your partner through either anger or seduction. Then I suggest that you each make a contract with the counselor to do your best not to do these things, no matter what.

Some examples of what Love Addicts might do to "anger bomb" their partners include denting the fender of the new car, "forgetting" to come home for two or three hours, charging up to or over the limit on one or more credit cards. The goal of such a maneuver is to make the partner angry enough to connect with the Love Addict in a fight, because at first even fighting is more comfortable than the quietness.

A common example of a Love Addict's "seduction bomb" is acting so helpless and childish that the partner feels compelled to connect with the Love Addict to take care of him or her. A second type of "seduction bomb" involves tantalizing sexual maneuvers to create intensity in the bedroom.

Some examples of a Love Avoidant's "anger bombs" might be threatening to leave, or becoming very judgmental and verbally attacking the partner with criticism about something the partner is doing. The goal is to trigger the partner's anger, compelling him or her to connect with the Love Avoidant with a fight.

Common examples of a Love Avoidant's "seduction bombs" might include offering to rescue the partner from difficulties, or inviting the partner on an exciting and romantic trip. A Love Avoidant might also use the other type of "seduction bomb" and make a passionate declaration to love the partner forever, or to entice and charm the Love Addict into being sexual with him or her, because Love Addicts often confuse sex with love; they often believe that when someone wants to be sexual with them, it is a crucial expression of true love.

WHAT TO DO WHEN THE
URGE TO BOMB ARISES

When you have an impulse to bomb through either anger or seduction, close your mouth and breathe. If all else fails, get up and leave the room. Love Addicts especially simply need to notice what is happening and not respond to it. This isn't as easy to do as it sounds, and there are some other things you can do inside your mind while you're restraining yourself.

I was helped through this by the instructions of my mentor, Janet Hurley. The following list is my own adaptation of her guidelines for me. When you follow these guidelines, you have a better chance of staying disengaged from your relationship, avoiding bombing or responding to your partner's bombs, and remaining in the withdrawal experience while you work on your own codependence and addiction recovery.[1]

1. Close your mouth and breathe.
2. Sit on your hands and repeat to yourself affirmations such as these:

   It is none of my business who my partner is.
   My partner has a right to be in this world the way he or she is.
   My job is to observe what is going on so that I can truly see who
   my partner is and respond in a mature way.
   My job is to take care of myself so I can be safe to my partner
   and be present for my relationship.

1These guidelines are available on six audio cassettes by Janet Hurley entitled "Recovery and Relationships" and available by writing Janet Hurley and Associates, P.O. Box 947, Carmel Valley, CA 93924.

My job is to refrain from hurting, punishing, attacking, getting even, fighting, or being dishonest.

3. Avoid getting reinvolved in the old addictive process of your relationship. For example, you might want to call somebody up and talk about how awful you think your partner is. Instead of doing that, sit still, meditate, and repeat an affirmation similar to this:

I have warm personal regard for my partner at all times.

If saying exactly these words seems so untrue that you have difficulty with them, keep in mind that it's important to have some affirmation about warm personal regard for your partner. Perhaps something like this will be more believable for you: "I have warm personal regard for all people at all times." Develop something along these lines about warm personal regard that feels authentic for you.

I added this phrase later on: "Although I hold this person in warm personal regard, I still have the right not to like some of his behavior or the problems that are created by this behavior." After a time of saying this, I felt relief from wanting to do the old destructive, addictive behaviors.

After a while you may find that your reaction to your partner's behavior is less toxic. The process leads you to learn to live with less reaction to what's going on. It also leads you to live with more action for yourself, as you keep yourself centered and unresponsive to what your partner is doing and saying that might trigger your addictive responses. The more you practice, the more you will be able to be in action for yourself, to be quiet, to be centered, and to be mature and appropriate. As a result you will become more "safe" to your partner, who may be rather frightened of being engulfed by your neediness.

4. Use a wall of pleasantness. While you are detaching and putting your relationship on hold, I strongly suggest that you practice good manners with this person and stop trying to get him or her to change or to hear you. Instead adopt a stance of simply observing and tracking what is happening.

Manners: No matter what, exercise the best manners you have around the other party, treating him or her as a very good friend. Don't react in anger, but rather focus on observing what is going on and remaining in an adult ego state. Show politeness and kindness, not irritation and misery. Sarcastic looks and condescending "courtesy" have *no* place in this approach.

Observation: Whenever there's any interaction, use the wall of pleasantness to deflect anything toxic that the person may send your way to get you upset. All the while pay close attention to what is going on. Since you have had an unrealistic fantasy of who your partner is, it's important to switch to being an active observer of who he or she really is, to listen to what the other party says about who he or she is.

This wall of pleasantness is in contrast to a destructive wall, such as a wall of silence or anger. With a destructive wall, you're blocking your partner out but also not seeing who he or she is. A wall of pleasantness means you are pleasant but very alert and observant of what's going on. Although you don't do much talking, you do say things that let your partner know you were listening. The other person experiences you as paying attention and feels valued and loved. It can really help calm the Love Avoidant's fear of being overwhelmed, engulfed, and controlled, and the Love Addict's fear of being abandoned.

The wall of pleasantness also "contains" you, restraining your impulsive tendency to crash into your partner's space with a hook of some sort. This pleasantness helps you resist beginning your abusive behavior. It can help you move from a position of wanting to attack your partner to a position of relative calm behind the wall of pleasantness.

You may feel somewhat phony using this wall, because in reality you may want to blast the partner. But think of it as a means for detaching from the addictive components of the relationship. Although this is not a healthy way to relate to anyone permanently, it can be a very necessary and helpful temporary part of recovery.

What often happens when you use this wall of pleasantness is that your partner may be pleasant in return. You may find that when this happens, you will like your partner a little better. As you use it, the wall of pleasantness may not feel as manipulative as it does at first, but more as if you are just being a reasonable person. The wall of pleasantness can often turn into a genuinely pleasant experience. And in many cases, when you become reasonable and pleasant, your partner may feel safer around you and more able to be present in the relationship.

WHAT CAN HELP YOU THROUGH WITHDRAWAL?

The next chapter describes additional helpful tools for Love Addicts, who usually experience more pain during the detachment phase of the recovery process than do Love Avoidants. Love Avoidants are not addicted to the partner, so the detachment does not bring up the same intensity of emotions. Love Avoidants can move to chapter 10, which describes recovery from codependence symptoms, although they might find it helpful to read chapter 9 in order to see what the Love Addict experiences as he or she wrestles with recovery.

9.

WITHDRAWING FROM
LOVE ADDICTION

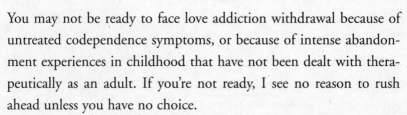

You may not be ready to face love addiction withdrawal because of untreated codependence symptoms, or because of intense abandonment experiences in childhood that have not been dealt with therapeutically as an adult. If you're not ready, I see no reason to rush ahead unless you have no choice.

You may have no choice because your partner has left and you must deal with the withdrawal experience. In this case facing these issues in the best way you can and doing some work on yourself can offer solid hope for entering another relationship (or resuming the relationship later, as in the case of a son, daughter, or parent) with more likelihood of fulfillment. But if you can do some codependence recovery and detoxification of childhood abandonment experiences first, before separating from your partner, then you can deal with the love addiction withdrawal more easily.

Reading this chapter can give you some idea of what to do with yourself if you're serious about going into withdrawal. If you're aware that you're not ready yet, you can use this section to begin to develop a game plan for when you are ready.

A Journaling Process for Facing Love Addiction

As with any other addiction, the following steps lead to withdrawal: breaking through denial to acknowledge your addiction, owning the harmful consequences, and then stepping in to intervene on the addictive cycle itself. I have developed journaling exercises for each of these steps. The specific journal exercise questions are given in chapters 14, 15, and 16. Below is a brief overview of the purpose of the questions and what they are about.

Acknowledging Your Addiction

The first exercise asks you to make a list of each person with whom you've experienced a co-addicted relationship. Begin with the first addictive relationship you can remember, which may have been with one of your parents, an older sister or brother, your first boyfriend or girlfriend, or your first counselor. End the list with the current relationship you're withdrawing from. Remember, while this person may be a sexual-romantic partner (spouse, lover), it may also be someone else, such as one of your children or one of your parents. Answer the set of questions for each person on your list.

The writing exercises guide you though describing (1) how you experienced each of the three love addiction symptoms; and (2) how you moved around the cycle of emotions experienced by Love Addicts, shown in Figure 1.

Facing Your Symptoms

Start with the first person on your list. Begin by describing how you assigned too much time, attention, and value above yourself, and made this person a Higher Power. Next describe your unrealistic expectations for this person to give you unconditional positive regard, and describe how this person couldn't do it because he or she abandoned (or is abandoning) the relationship with an addiction. Continue with the next person, until you have completed your list.

As you write you will probably be able to move toward accepting the fact that while you can get pretty close to giving yourself unconditional positive regard, nobody else can really do that for you, whether they are involved in an addiction or not, because they're human beings. You will be guided to write in your own words an acknowledgment that there are few people, if any, who can consistently give you unconditional positive regard.

Then, if it is one of your symptoms, you will write about how you stopped taking care of yourself and valuing yourself when you got into a co-addictive relationship with somebody.

Recognizing Your Movement Through the Emotional Cycle

The writing then helps you identify how you were attracted to the other person, felt high as your childhood fantasy was triggered, and denied the reality of who the person was. The questions take you through the rest of the emotional cycle for Love Addicts, as shown in Figure 1: how the reality finally did come clear, how awful you felt, how the person abandoned the relationship, what planning you did to get that person back into the relationship, how you acted out your plan or plans, what happened, and how you cycled around again, either in a new relationship or with the same person. You also track how the positive and negative intensity happened to you.

This process helps you into the first stage of addiction recovery —breaking through denial. "This is how I do it. I've done it several (or many) times. Hey, I've got the symptoms!"

Entering a Grieving Process

Acknowledging that few people can consistently give unconditional positive regard usually throws people into a grieving process, so don't be surprised if it happens to you. With these words you surrender your painkiller, the equivalent of the bottle to the alcoholic. Your "bottle" is your desire for unconditional positive regard from another person. Your acknowledgment that you probably aren't going to get consistent unconditional positive regard from anyone parallels the alcoholic's acknowledgment that the bottle isn't really going to make him or her feel better over the long haul. Writing about this leads you to surrender some of your skewed thinking, which is the doorway to actually intervening on the addiction.

Examining Harmful Consequences

The next step in arresting love addiction is to examine any harmful consequences that have occurred as a result of your love addiction.

Here are a few other serious harmful consequences I have gleaned from Love Addicts who have shared with me as they began to face their lives. Perhaps they will help you get in touch with your own particular set of harmful consequences:

- Abandoning your children for the person to whom you are addicted. Love Addict parents can become so obsessed by and compulsive about an adult Love Avoidant that they do not want to spend time with their children, pay attention to them, or do things for them. The person they are addicted to takes priority over everything, and Love Addicts would rather obsess about that person than be a parent.
- Having a series of relationships, or even marriages, and not being able to sustain one over a long period of time.
- Living with and setting yourself up for intense emotions

(highs and lows) on a daily basis—rarely having a sense of peace and serenity or of being comfortable with oneself.

- Having little or no intimate relationship with your adult children because of continually focusing on the object of your love addiction.
- Never having married because of being love-addicted to a parent and thus being unable to form a romantic relationship.
- Either not getting help for psychological problems, or getting abused in therapy because of being addicted to a counselor.
- Being love-addicted to a child and losing a romantic relationship.
- Nearly getting arrested for having beaten up somebody who was in a sexual affair with your partner.
- Being love-addicted to a physically abusive person and allowing yourself or your children to be beaten up or otherwise seriously abused.
- Being love addicted to a sex addict who is an incest perpetrator; knowing that and yet staying with the person and allowing your daughter or son to be an incest victim.

Examining Your Participation in Each Stage of the Cycle

The journaling process next leads you to consider the chronic progressive stages of love addiction that were described in chapter 3. You will write about how you've done these stages, and determine which stage you are currently experiencing at this time.

Fantasy, Emotional High, Relief from Pain

This section of the journaling guidelines examines the initial attraction, the way the love or rescue fantasy that you developed in childhood is activated, and the high experience that brings relief from the pain of codependence, all of which are described in chapter 3.

It is important to realize that during the fantasy phase, your contact with some aspects of reality almost doesn't exist. A closer look taken in this journaling process at the real person you were viewing as a knight in shining armor or a super-female rescuer reveals that he or she was far less perfect than you could see at the time. Seeing this person as a rescuing figure was fantasy.

I've found it very helpful to write about where you are in these various stages of the addiction. How chronic is your love addiction? This analysis helps you explore even more thoroughly the harmful consequences of your love addiction.

Stopping the Cycles: Intervention and Withdrawal

After journaling through these issues, you probably have enough information to intervene on your love addiction. At this point you disengage from the addictive part of your relationship, as described in chapter 8.

It is at this time that some Love Addicts may need physician-prescribed antidepressant medication to moderate the impulse to self-harm that may be caused by the intense pain, fear, and rage that come up during withdrawal. Their intense fear can lead to panic attacks, and intense rage can turn homicidal. Medications that are not highly psychoactive are appropriate for people who are chemically dependent. Such medications relieve the intense emotional experience just enough to allow the Love Addict to do the work of recovery. Such antidepressants are used only for a short time, usually averaging about three months.

Detoxification from History of Abandonment

While you, the Love Addict, are in withdrawal, cycling through pain, fear, anger, and emptiness, I recommend working with a counselor who can teach you how to "discover" (recover) your childhood history of abandonment. (It is my strong opinion that any kind of child abuse is an abandonment experience.) The counselor can help you journal about the specific relevant details, and then guide you through the process of talking about what happened, allowing you to own and release the old childhood emotions about the abandonment.

A Review of Current Walls

Next you will need to look at the nuts and bolts of how you are being avoided currently by your Love Avoidant. Look at how your partner has avoided you by staying behind walls. You will probably cycle through intense grieving, not only about how your original caregivers abandoned and abused you but also about how your partner in your current relationship has avoided you. It may take from six to twelve months to do all this work, and during that process it is not unusual for a Love Addict to feel very lonely.

I thought I was going through the darkest days of my life during this experience; but on the exterior, unbeknownst to me, I was going through a phenomenal positive change. Other people noticed physical signs: They let me know that my facial expression had become softer and more relaxed, and my voice sounded less angry. Their comments let me know how destructive the toxic effects of such serious abandonment and abuse can be for us.

WORKING ON CORE SYMPTOMS OF CODEPENDENCE

During this time you, as a Love Addict, need to work through an inventory of how you experience the fourth core symptom of codependence: difficulty meeting your own needs and wants. The journal guideline provides a place for you to inventory all the needs that heretofore you have not taken care of adequately. You will examine such needs as sexual needs, financial needs, food issues, and physical nurture, to name a few.

As you progress in recovery, you can begin to take responsibility for meeting your needs in a healthy and positive way. Perhaps you need to contact a financial planner. You may start doing something new with any sexual issues you may have, or do some work in terms of getting physical nurture. And you can begin to address any other addictions you recognize, such as an eating addiction or spending addiction. Each of your needs, and the ways you try to meet them, interplays with the other.

The experience of recovery from love addiction has brought me the most incredible pain I've faced in my recovery journey, but facing this addiction is still the most wonderful thing I ever did for myself. Pain is not the enemy; the fear of passing through pain is. And I want to encourage you to begin because of my experience and my strong belief that you can stand it. After all, it's only your pain, and you can learn to tolerate your own pain.

10.

TREATING THE SYMPTOMS OF CODEPENDENCE

As we've seen, the core symptoms of codependence are the ways in which our relationship with ourself fails, creating internal pain that drives us to one or more addictive processes. By healing each core symptom, we begin to establish increasing levels of internal comfort. This greatly alleviates both the drive toward addictive processes and the secondary symptoms described in chapter 1.

Recovery from codependence involves two separate processes: treating the primary and secondary symptoms, and treating the cause. The cause is child abuse, a toxic experience for a child that creates chronic stress past childhood into adulthood. You need to detoxify from the chronic stress by going back in your mind and looking at what happened, exploring how you felt about it both as a child and today as an adult. After that you also need to look at the harmful consequences that those traumatic experiences create in your adult life today.

As you embark upon your recovery from codependence, it's important to keep in mind whether you are working on recovery from one of the codependent symptoms, or treating the toxic effects of how you were abused as a child. These are two distinct processes that need to be kept separate.

TREATING THE CAUSE

Treating the toxic effects from your personal history involves getting educated about what abuse is, writing about your own abuse history, and going through a psychological detoxification process. A person usually experiences detoxification in a group with guidance and support from a counselor. The counselor guides the person to do two things: (1) to claim the feelings about what happened in childhood—both the adult feelings now and the old child feelings; and (2) to claim and modify any existing immature, toxic, childish thinking or behavior still present in the adult codependent.

To claim our feelings about abusive childhood experiences, we use words such as, "This is what happened to me, and today as an adult I have these adult feelings about it; when I was a child I had these child feelings." We need to release all that toxic energy from the child part of ourselves. It is in those very simple statements and the willingness to reexperience the old feeling reality and have our present-day feelings about it that we detoxify from the effects of that old trauma. Then we enter a grieving process, grieving the losses of our childhood.

To modify any existing immature childish thinking, it is helpful to let a counselor, sponsor, or trusted recovering friend point out such thinking when they hear it. After having it pointed out a few times, we become able to notice our own immature thinking and begin to correct it by doing some non-shaming self-talk about what a more mature, realistic way of thinking about an issue in question would be. Some of the more common examples of immature childish toxic thinking that I hear from Love Addicts include, "Someday, someone will provide me with everything my parents didn't give me," "Life should be fair," and "I can't stand it."

Treating the Primary and Secondary Symptoms

Most of us need instruction and help as we deal with our primary symptoms. We need to learn or relearn how to value ourselves (self-esteem), develop boundaries, identify who we are and share that appropriately, take care of our needs and wants interdependently, and become centered and moderate.

Although the secondary symptoms strongly resist recovery before the primary symptoms have been addressed, they can be improved upon after some healing of the primary symptoms has taken place. We begin to be able to find ways to stop negative control; to deal with issues of injustice in some way besides resentment, recycling old anger, and getting even; to become a spiritual person, however we define it; to refrain from using addictions or physical or mental illness to avoid reality; and to become able to be intimate.

There is an end to codependence treatment—it isn't something one does forever. Three to five years is the average, although most people find a continuing Twelve-Step journey helpful to prevent relapsing into the old wagon-ruts of codependent behaviors.

Stages of Recovery from Codependence

As work on these areas of recovery progresses, people usually pass through different stages of healing from both the childhood issues and the adult symptoms. As long as you are still functioning at any of these levels, I strongly suggest that you not reenter your relationship or start a new one. Here is a brief review of these stages.

1. Denial

About childhood: "I was not abused as a child."

About adult life: "I am not a codependent."

2. Blaming the Offender

About childhood: "I admit I was abused, but it's all my parent's fault. If they don't get well, I can't."

About adult life: "I have codependence, but I can't get well until my partner does. It is all your (the partner's) fault I am sick anyway. I wouldn't be codependent if I weren't in a relationship with you. If I had a healthy person to relate to, I wouldn't be acting this way."

Although we are not to *blame* others for our inability to recover, we do need to face the reality of what was done to us and hold accountable those whose behavior harmed us.

3. Accountability

About childhood: "I am now able to hold my major caregiver accountable for what was done to me, and I have my feelings about what happened to me in childhood." (We have moved into co-dependence recovery regarding the childhood abuse issues when we can make such a statement.)

About adult life: "I hold myself responsible for my codependence and recovery from the symptoms."

At this point a few people are ready to reenter their relationship, but most are still not.

4. Survival

During this stage you can probably begin to reenter your relationship.

About childhood: "I am beginning to feel relief from my feelings about the childhood abuse as I let go of the intense emotions surrounding what happened to me." (It is probably at this point that you can start making requests for intimacy and support from the partner with whom you are reestablishing a relationship.)

About adult life: "I am beginning to experience a sense of personal power and hope as I heal from my dysfunction and self-defeating symptoms and take charge of my life."

When you reach stage four regarding your adult life, you have developed some skill at self-care and are not so dependent on your partner. Now, whether you are a Love Addict or an Love Avoidant, you can reenter your relationship.

5. Integration

This stage is the same for both the childhood issues and the adult symptoms: "I now see that what happened to me has created who I am. I'm grateful because I see how the problems created by the abuse have in turn created my spiritual path and given me some depth of character and wisdom."

FIVE CONCURRENT PROCESSES IN RECOVERY FROM THE CO-ADDICTED RELATIONSHIP

Five recovery processes are interwoven during the healing of a co-addicted relationship. Recovery begins with number one and develops through five, but one or more may occur simultaneously. In my opinion it is unwise to reenter a relationship prematurely; but at the same time you don't want to let recovery go on so long that you don't get back to the work of the relationship. So, just to give some idea of when working on the relationship is safe and appropriate, I want to describe the five processes and indicate where you can probably reenter the relationship.

1. Growing Up

This process involves confronting the five primary symptoms of the illness and beginning a healing process from them. It includes learning how to have self-esteem, boundaries, a sense of self, self-care, and moderation.

2. Facing Reality

This process begins as soon as you have begun to confront and heal the third primary symptom, difficulty owning your own reality. Facing reality means taking a look at who you are and who others are. I wouldn't suggest entering or reentering a relationship here; this part of the process of facing reality may involve looking at one's partner and saying, "Let me out of here." Although your first response to a realistic view of the partner may be to break away, after doing further recovery work for yourself (especially increased maturity, improved boundaries, and greater ability at self-care), your partner's flaws may not seem so devastating.

3. Grieving Losses

Grieving losses means having feelings about what you lost in childhood and what the disease has cost you in adulthood. In between this and the next process, you could probably reenter the relationship, especially after you have done sufficient grieving.

4. Learning to Reparent Yourself

Learning to reparent yourself begins when you begin to work on the fourth core symptom, difficulty meeting your own needs and wants. This process involves learning how to affirm yourself, nurture yourself, and limit yourself without shaming yourself.

5. Learning to Forgive

Forgiveness means giving up the desire to have abusive people in your life sufficiently punished. This fifth process involves both forgiveness of yourself for the costs of the disorder, and forgiveness of major care-givers for what happened. Some abuse is so terrible that the issue of forgiveness probably should not be broached unless the person who is the victim brings it up. If you have been an offender and abused someone, I recommend that you work on self-forgiveness and for-giveness from your Higher Power first. Asking the victim for forgive-ness probably needs to wait until that person brings it up. I realize that this seems to contradict traditional religious training, but when dealing with severe abuse situations, an offender's premature request for the victim's forgiveness may only aggravate the victim's situation so that the offender can feel better.

CORRECTING DISTORTED THINKING:
THE LOVE ADDICT

Love Addicts who confront symptom number three—difficulty own-ing your own reality—need to confront several distorted attitudes or beliefs. One dominant attitude Love Addicts need to revamp is that of expecting warm personal regard and caretaking from someone all the time. While this expectation is reasonable for a child, it is not realistic for adults. As codependence recovery progresses, you adjust your thinking to accept the fact that you are fortunate to get warm personal regard from somebody some of the time. In recovery you begin to notice that this happens most often when your genuine self is also who your partner wants you to be. It also happens when your value system about something naturally coincides with your partner's value system, and therefore your partner is comfortable and you are not diminished. In recovery from love addiction, however, you no longer reshape or recolor your reality to get the approval or warm regard.

Love Addicts need to accept the fact that other people may not like their choices or thinking or feeling reality. In recovery you understand that you will probably not get warm personal regard when your way of being or of doing something conflicts with another person's value system or the way that other person wants you to be. However healthy such a choice may be for you, if others must give up or do without a level of comfort because of this choice, it is unlikely that they will like it—even though they may accept it out of respect for your right to live your own life. With healthy boundaries you just know that, expect it, and still go on to be who you are, giving up the unrealistic expectation that the other person will like everything about you.

Working toward healing the first and fourth symptoms of codependence (difficulty experiencing appropriate self-esteem and difficulty taking care of the self) will greatly assist you to make this important attitude shift. In recovery the most important person in your life who can give you consistent warm personal regard is yourself. You focus on generating warm personal regard from within because you have experienced a degree of healing for that first core symptom of codependence—difficulty with self-esteem. Your growing ability to be responsible for your own needs and wants also enhances your ability to go ahead and be your authentic self with greater assurance that your needs and wants will be met, even if other people in your life withdraw their support. With recovery in the area of self-esteem and self-care, you can begin to move away from attempting to enmesh with your partner and learn healthy intimacy.

For example, a busy wife may choose to tell the family that she will no longer take the time to search through the pockets of the dirty clothes to remove personal articles before washing the clothes, or to turn clothes right side out before she puts them in the washing machine. The members of the family must make sure their own pockets are empty—or expect to have the contents of the pockets put through the wash. They may make sure the clothes are right side out before they put them in the hamper, or find them returned clean but still inside out. They may understand her reasons, and even accept their new responsibilities. But they may not like the extra work or the drenched billfolds that come back to them when they forget to check their pockets. The wife, while noticing that the family complains about her decision, can still feel comfortable about her choice and hold herself in warm personal regard. She has not done anything "wrong" just because the family doesn't like what she has decided. And she has taken responsibility for her own need to be less busy by spreading more of the responsibility for the housework among the other family members.

Here's another example. James, who is a Love Addict in relationship to his mother, wants to be a teacher. His mother has her heart set on James being a lawyer so he can earn lots of money. She does not like it that James has completed a Ph.D. degree and accepted a teaching job in a small private college. While James has the right to choose his own career, he needs to accept that his mother is not happy about his choice. These instances of conflict in value systems, or one person's natural behavior causing discomfort for the other, are common occurrences in close relationships. James is not doing anything "wrong" simply because his mother doesn't like his vocational choice. In recovery James takes responsibility for his desire to be a teacher and can be very comfortable with who he is, while simply being aware that his mother does not like his career choice.

A second point of distorted thinking recovering Love Addicts need to adjust is to stop regarding any other person as all-important, all-powerful, and perfect—or a Higher Power. All people are perfectly imperfect, and are of equal value. Making progress in healing the first symptom of codependence, experiencing appropriate levels of self-esteem, greatly assists the recovering Love Addict to adjust this view.

A third attitude shift Love Addicts need to make is away from the concept that someone else will take care of them. Again, this is appropriate for a child, but as adults we are each responsible for seeing that our own needs and wants are being met. Recovery in the fourth core symptom of codependence is a great asset in renovating this dysfunctional attitude toward healthy self-care.

CORRECTING DISTORTED THINKING: THE LOVE AVOIDANT

Several inappropriate attitudes need to be adjusted as a Love Avoidant begins to work with core symptom number three, difficulty owning one's own reality. One major view that needs correcting is a faulty concept of intimacy. Because they experienced emotional-sexual abuse (either overt or covert) as a child, Love Avoidants learned that to be intimate means someone will enmesh with them, transgress their boundaries, and in the process Love Avoidants will lose their sense of self. Healthy intimacy is simply sharing one's reality with another and receiving the reality of another, with each person having boundaries so that neither enmeshment nor other forms of abuse can happen. Working toward healing in the second and third core symptoms of codependence (difficulty setting boundaries and difficulty owning one's own reality) is very effective in helping the Love Avoidant straighten out this inaccurate concept of intimacy.

As we've seen, Love Avoidants do not readily share intimate details about their thoughts, feelings, needs, or wants, for fear that the other person will use this information to manipulate or control them into caretaking. Many Love Avoidants have even lost touch with their own reality in one or more areas, and don't know what they feel or think about many things. After Love Avoidants have made progress with healing the third symptom of codependence, difficulty knowing one's own reality, they find it easier to get in touch with their own reality. Once in touch with their true thoughts and feelings, for instance, recovering Love Avoidants can then learn how to share their reality appropriately with someone. Also, with healthy boundaries, they can share such information with better assurance that good boundaries can prevent their being controlled or manipulated by someone trying to make use of the information.

In addition, after Love Avoidants have progressed in developing healthy boundaries, they find that receiving someone else's reality is less toxic. Recovering Love Avoidants can either resonate with this data or notice it but choose to block it from further consideration and just be aware that the other person has that reality. With healthy boundaries the recovering person does not get overwhelmed or controlled by the reality of the other person and let it trigger irrational fears or obsessive thoughts. (When dealing with a "major offender," however, healthy boundaries usually do not provide enough protection and it becomes appropriate to use walls. See *Facing Codependence*, pages 11–21.)

This kind of recovery and change is made more difficult when the partner is still an active Love Addict. The Love Addict partner is attempting to enmesh, and probably will use intimate information to try to manipulate and control. So part of the problem the Love Avoidant has in trying to be intimate with the partner is truly about the partner.

Another distorted belief of Love Avoidants is that their job is to take care of the partner, and that if the Love Avoidant doesn't do this job, the other party will not be interested in a relationship. In a healthy relationship it is not one's job to take care of another adult. Each of us is responsible for our own self-care.

Further, Love Avoidants need to make adjustments regarding being adored. It is not appropriate to be in a position in which another person sees them as all-important, all-powerful, all-perfect.

Many Love Avoidants believe that a needy, dependent person is a safe person who can be controlled. This belief needs to be adjusted: A needy, dependent person is not safe. Such a person can drain the partner, wanting the partner to parent him or her and meet most or all personal needs. Therefore, being attracted to such a person and entering a relationship with one is dangerous—that is, not safe. The key here is to realize that one uses boundaries to create safety for the self in a relationship, not relying on the diminished capacity of someone else and the potential for control over that person.

In addition, Love Avoidants tend to be unable to take care of themselves when faced with a dependent person demonstrating neediness. Love Avoidants usually take care of the other person to the detriment of themselves. This often leads to resentment, which is then used to justify acting out in an addiction outside the relationship. Working toward healing in these core symptoms of codependence can help reverse this process, making it possible for recovering Love Avoidants to be in action for themselves and allow the partner to find other resources when the recovering Love Avoidants cannot give care to the partner without diminishing themselves.

Also needing adjustment is the belief of many Love Avoidants that a person who displays vulnerability is worth less or has less value than the Love Avoidant. To use the natural characteristics of a person to label that person as less-than is part of the disease of codependence. Developing healing in the first core symptom—experiencing appropriate levels of self-esteem—can move a recovering Love Avoidant's thinking toward the realization that nobody has less or more value than anyone else in terms of inherent worth.

LEARNING TO ACCEPT ANOTHER'S VALUE SYSTEM

Until I began to recover with regard to all five symptoms of co-dependence—learning self-esteem, setting my boundaries, identifying who I am, taking care of myself, and doing it all with greater moderation—it was difficult to tolerate experiences of conflict between my husband's values and mine. I wanted to change his values so that I could be comfortable and have a partner who operated in a manner that fit my values.

My husband grew up an Irish Catholic and I grew up a German Protestant. Parts of his value system are very different from mine, and I have difficulty accepting them. Of course, he looks at the way I operate in my German Protestant habits and thinks I'm kind of strange, too. So what does that mean? It just means that we have different values.

A value, or belief, is related to how we think the world is supposed to work and how we are supposed to behave. When we are operating outside our own values, or breaking our own rules, we feel guilt. When our partner requires us to operate outside our values, the result is conflict: guilt for ourselves if we comply with the partner's requirement, or disruption within the relationship if we refuse.

An example of a values conflict between a couple might be when one approves of abortion and the other doesn't. Another example could be that one partner believes in living off of credit, and the other believes one should only buy with cash. One person may believe that expensive cosmetics are really helpful and advantageous, and the other thinks that they are ridiculous and a waste of money. Another conflict many couples deal with is over time: One person might believe that when you don't keep your time agreements, you're being irresponsible; the other might believe timeliness isn't that important and often arrives late to appointments.

When a person has established a set of values—belief about how the world should work and how one should conduct oneself in it—and sees someone else operating outside these values, he or she often becomes critical and judgmental and may see the other person as being bad or less-than. The person doing the critical judging is operating in his or her codependence. In recovery, especially in relationship recovery, it's important to recognize our partner's value system and stop trying to get our partner to change it if it is not actually abusive to us. Instead, we need to allow our partner to operate within the partner's own value system, while we also operate within our own. Values are usually not very negotiable and are not that easily changed, especially in the important areas of money, sex, abortion, and other life issues.

It may be possible, however, that certain values are in such great conflict that they become a good reason for terminating a relationship. Let's say Sally, a Love Addict, married Kirk. The reality of Kirk's values was not apparent at the time, because Sally was operating out of fantasy, thinking the values of her fantasy hero were Kirk's values. In recovery Sally discovers that Kirk's value system really runs counter to her own in some major areas. He may be a thief, a rapist, or a physical abuser "behind closed doors."

This could happen to Kirk as well. Sally, a Love Addict, would work hard in the beginning to present herself to Kirk in a way that Kirk would find pleasing, so she would probably withhold from Kirk any information about her differing values. As recovery progresses Sally begins to be more honest about her values, and Kirk discovers that her values run counter to his. Since Kirk can only be comfortable operating within his value system, and Sally can only be comfortable operating within hers, there is not a whole lot of room to resolve this issue. Resolution requires one of them to shift his or her values, and that is hard to do.

Addiction recovery, however, requires value modification. A sex addict places a high value on sex, an alcoholic places a high value on drinking, a spending addict places a high value on living off of credit, and so forth. To the extent that the person's value of the item addicted to can be modified so that the addict can refrain from being obsessive and compulsive about whatever it is, recovery can take place. So if both people are in recovery, it is prudent to wait to see what changes occur as a result of recovery from any addiction before deciding if a partner's differing value system around the addiction issue is truly incompatible or tolerable.

This kind of value modification by both parties and the acceptance of the newly discovered values of the other is another area in which we need codependence recovery before we can experience the maturity necessary to heal from either set of symptoms that make up the two parts of a co-addicted relationship.

11.

ENTERING OR REENTERING
A RELATIONSHIP

I believe that the primary purpose of relationships is to allow two people to be connected to each other through intimacy, so that each gets support from the other to ease the burdens of life and to enhance the enjoyment of living. The maturity level we need to maintain a healthy relationship is reflected by having a sense of self-esteem, the ability to set boundaries, a good sense of self, improved self-care, and the ability to share who we are moderately (and in appropriate ways and at appropriate times) with our partners. In other words, recovery from the core symptoms of codependence is necessary for a mature and enhancing intimate relationship.

This next phase of recovery involves reentering the relationship. In recovery, we enter a relationship with requests for two things: intimacy and support. Each request needs to be verbal, direct, and clear to the partner. At the same time, we listen to and respond to our partner's requests for intimacy and support.

REQUESTS FOR INTIMACY

Intimacy means sharing and receiving reality without judgment. We can share three forms of reality: our body, thoughts, and feelings.

Sharing Your Body

We can engage in two forms of intimacy with the body: to exchange physical contact, and to exchange sexual contact.

Physical intimacy includes a wide range of physical contact that shows affection and concern without creating sexual arousal. Its purpose is to comfort the partner or the self. Some examples are holding hands, hugging, touching feet under the covers while going to sleep, giving or receiving a back rub or neck rub.

You might phrase a direct request for physical intimacy like this: "Would you be willing to give me a hug? Would you be willing to hold my hand?"

The request is not, "May I hug you?" but "Will you hug me?" This is a request to have your partner initiate the intimacy by giving the hug. Knowing what boundaries are and having developed them, a recovering person negotiates these experiences through this use of the external boundary system.

Sexual intimacy includes sharing the body in sexual ways, and its purpose is to create sexual arousal. You might phrase a request for sexual intimacy like this: "Would you be willing to be sexual with me tonight?"

Sharing Your Thoughts

Intellectual intimacy is sharing your thoughts with your partner or listening to your partner's thoughts. An important aspect of intellectual intimacy is to know and say clearly that the content of what you are sharing is your own thinking and not necessarily the way things are. To make requests for intellectual intimacy, you might say something like, "I need to talk to you about this, would you be willing to talk about this with me?" Or you might phrase the request like this: "Would you be willing to meet me for breakfast at seven o'clock in the morning so we can discuss what we're going to do about remodeling the kitchen?" Or you might say, "I've been thinking about an idea to give us more privacy separate from the kids. Would you be willing to talk with me about it?"

Sharing Your Feelings

Emotional intimacy is revealing your emotions or listening while someone else expresses his or hers. Often intellectual and emotional intimacy go together. As we disclose our thoughts, the feelings connected to them also become known.

You might phrase requests for emotional intimacy like this: "Would you be willing to listen while I share some feelings I have about what just happened?" or "Would you be willing to tell me what you're experiencing emotionally about what just happened?"

REQUESTS FOR SUPPORT

Asking for support means asking your partner to help meet a need or want. To do that directly, you might say something like, "I want to go see this movie tonight. Would you be willing to go with me?" A request for support for a physical need might be, "Would you be willing to look at my finger and try to remove this splinter?" Other examples of requests for support with a physical need might include asking someone to scratch your back, give your neck a massage, or bandage a small wound you can't reach yourself.

A request for emotional support might be, "Would you be willing to go with me to see my son graduate? I want emotional support from you while I'm around my ex-husband and all his family." A request for support with the need for time, attention, and direction might be, "Would you be willing to give me some direction around this business problem I'm having?" or "Would you go shopping with me? I want you to see what this outfit looks like and give me feedback I will use to decide whether to buy it or not."

SOME GUIDELINES TO FOLLOW AFTER MAKING REQUESTS

If you participated in a co-addicted relationship, you were trying to relate to people with behavior patterns that didn't work. These behavior patterns were designed to find ways to force your partner to meet your needs and be intimate with you. Now, as a recovering person, you begin making specific requests—not so much to make someone meet your needs, but to make your needs known—while leaving room for the person to choose whether or not to respond to your need. The next step is to learn what to do after the request is made.

These guidelines from my friend and mentor, Janet Hurley, taught me some healthy behavior to replace the manipulative, controlling things I had done before. They helped me so much that I offer them to you, along with how I interpreted them, as helpful rules to follow when you're tempted to go back to old behavior patterns.

1. Show Up
Up until now the relationship was on hold. Now you reenter the relationship by being physically in the presence of the other person more. Make your presence in the relationship a priority as opposed to making your individual treatment and recovery the only priority.

For example, if a couple had made a decision to physically separate, "showing up" might mean moving back together again. If they had continued to live in the same house, "showing up" might mean going out to dinner regularly.

2. Pay Attention
When in your partner's presence, actively listen to what your partner tells you about what is happening to him or her.

3. Tell the Truth
At this point you need to be rigorously honest. This doesn't mean being completely open, because it is often not helpful. It is in your best interest to refrain from sharing certain things. While your partner does not need to know all about you, you do tell the truth concerning those things you choose to share. In your therapy you can ask for the help you need to figure out what data needs to be private. When your partner requests information that you don't want to give, but you also don't want to lie, you simply say, "I'm not willing to discuss that." This, too, is the truth.

4. Ask for What You Need and Want
Make clear requests for intimacy and support. Reveal what you need or what you want, and what you would like your partner to do to help you take care of that need or want.

5. Let Go of Attachment to the Outcome
When you make requests for intimacy or support from your partner, let go of any emotional investment in the answer. The point of making the request is identifying and asking for what you need and want from your partner. This enables you to practice revealing what you want without the hidden, devious, veiled methods that were hard to comprehend and so often the cause of misunderstandings. No matter how your partner responds, your attitude should be, "So this is my partner's response today. Isn't it interesting?"

A clear "no" to your request is not necessarily a rejection of you as a person; it is an indication that the other person is not willing to do the specific thing you requested at this time. Understanding this distinction is necessary for recovery in the relationship.

I realize that this is difficult, but it keeps the focus off of the need to control or manipulate your partner into giving you what you want. I found it took a lot of courage for me just to present a simple request and stand back.

6. Learn to Celebrate Your Partner's "No"

When you make a request for intimacy or support and the answer is "no," you learn to be content or even happy with that. As maturity develops you become able to accept that your partner may have to say no at times in the interest of his or her own self-care. You can learn not to take this as a personal rejection and celebrate the fact that your partner is taking care of himself or herself, even though it isn't especially helpful to you. You can accept and celebrate that fact because you're taking such good care of yourself now. You're in codependence recovery, addressing the fourth primary symptom, and have learned how to take care of your needs and wants interdependently. You have others in your life that you can go to for help and support and for intimacy. You're not so dependent on your partner.

7. Note What You Get

Instead of making sure your request is answered with a "yes," or confronting your partner with the request again and again because you don't like his or her response, just keep an inventory of what the requests are, how many "no" answers you get, and how many "yes" answers you get.

Keeping this inventory helps to answer the question, "How am I going to know whether to stay in this relationship or leave it?" You'll know by tracking whether there are enough "yes" responses to make the relationship satisfying for you. It is an individual choice, and it's nobody's business how you make that choice. Many relationships today have more to do with support than survival. It's probably not very wise to stay in a relationship that is extremely unsupportive. In some cases, however, because some of us have such serious abandonment issues, there may be exceptions. Some Love Addicts have had such severe experiences of abuse that it may be better for them to stay with a dysfunctional partner than to be alone. The only time I question someone is if violent physical, sexual, or verbal abuse is going on, especially when there are children in the home.

If we have friends who are in very unsupportive relationships, or when we as counselors treat such people, it is very important not to encourage them to leave, or even to say such things as, "Well, there's something terribly wrong with you that you would stay with this person. Anyone in their right mind would leave." That is inappropriate. It's none of our business what this person needs to live with. We have no idea whether it would be worse for that person to leave and be alone, or at least to have someone else in the house.

I've found that trying to inventory "yes" and "no" responses before you begin codependence recovery is not very helpful. As you improve your ability to take care of your own needs and wants and feel comfortable owning that responsibility, you need less from your partner, and the "no" answers you get don't bother you as much.

Another common pitfall—one I experienced—is that before codependence recovery we tend to keep track of the "no" answers and ignore the "yes" answers. They don't even make it to our inventory! Our partners notice this because they can see that we come to the wrong conclusions frequently. We tell them, "You never compliment me" or "You never do anything with me that I like to do. It's always what you want to do." But your partner may actually be saying "yes" more frequently than you think.

For example, one person asks the partner to be more intentional about giving compliments. When the partner responds with a compliment a few days later, the person can easily negate it mentally. Let's say Jed tells his roommate, Kent, that he really likes the way Kent has arranged the living room furniture. Kent listens, but thinks, "Jed is just saying that because I asked him to give more compliments. It's obvious to me the living room still needs adjusting before it's really right," thereby negating Jed's compliment. Jed is doing what Kent asked him to do: looking for something he can honestly affirm and giving a sincere compliment. But Kent's thinking process makes it possible for him to ignore the fact that Jed has affirmed him.

It's even possible to make a "yes" into a "no" if we think about it long enough. I remember having perfectly good supportive experiences that, by the time they were over, seemed to me to be some of the worst abandonment experiences I'd ever had. If our childhood experiences of abandonment are severe enough, we start looking for abandonment in every corner.

An example of turning a "yes" into a "no" might happen in this way. Let's say Sara asks her brother, Bob, to go visit their Aunt Jessie while he is on a trip to Denver. Bob has never gotten along with Aunt Jessie, but he agrees to go, adding that he will be uncomfortable doing it. Susan then gets angry and says, "Well, just don't go, then! I don't want you to go anyway." Instead of accepting Bob's "yes" but allowing him to have his discomfort about it, Susan turned his "yes" into a "no."

RESPONDING TO YOUR PARTNER'S
REQUESTS FOR INTIMACY AND SUPPORT

The other side of this process is to learn to evaluate when and how to respond to your partner's requests. When your partner makes requests of you, it is sometimes difficult to figure out whether you should or shouldn't respond. What criteria do we use if we're no longer people-pleasing or if we're trying to take responsibility for our own self-care? What is a reasonable way to determine how to respond? Here's a rule of thumb I use: Say yes when responding is not too great a cost for you; say no when the cost will be too great.

For example, your partner may ask you to be sexual, and you're a little tired. It will take some effort to get into it. But it's important to take care of the relationship, and you're willing to put forth some effort to do it. Being sexual only when you're absolutely comfortable doing it usually doesn't work out, because after a sexual-romantic relationship has existed for a while, waiting for both people to be absolutely comfortable and interested in sex at the same time means that too few opportunities for sex occur. So there are times when responding may require compromising your ideal wishes for the moment.

If you have to compromise so far that you hurt yourself, however, then you need to refuse. For example, your partner might request that you be sexual, but you have a stomach virus and are nauseous. It would be very uncomfortable for you to have sex with your partner, and a refusal would be appropriate. In more subtle situations, this kind of awareness usually takes some work and practice to develop.

GUIDELINES FOR BEING IN A RELATIONSHIP

Here are some guidelines Pat and I have developed for our own relationship that we find very helpful, especially when we're discussing something or sharing our intellectual and emotional reality with each other.

1. Don't Assign Blame When You're in Conflict
When you confront your partner about something, don't make your partner wrong. Just make statements about what happened and what feelings you're having about it. I find that this takes a lot of discipline.

Make sure the statement about what you perceived happening does not include any hidden or open message about the other person being less-than. For example, it implies the person is less-than to say, "When you were acting like a nincompoop in the garage . . ." A more appropriate statement might be, "Yesterday, when you walked into the garage and raised your voice to a high volume and said . . ." Describe what happened without labeling the person a nincompoop.

2. Don't Keep Score on Your Partner

When your partner is confronting you about your behavior, avoid bringing up how the partner did the same thing several times last week. What your partner did last week is not relevant to the conversation this week. The two of you are discussing what you've done this week.

3. Don't Argue Perceptions (or Facts)

Understand that each partner has perceptions, and your job is to identify your own perception and listen to your partner's perception. We can probably be most respectful of our partner simply by hearing who that person is without judgment or trying to make our partner change his or her reality.

For example, let's say you and your best friend, Elizabeth, are looking at a turtle. You say, "What a nice color green!" And Elizabeth responds, "No, it's more blue than green." Once you are aware that the turtle looks blue to Elizabeth, don't try to argue her into saying that it's green. Letting Elizabeth have her own reality makes her feel your love. You keep your perception of the green turtle and let it go. At first this may seem like dishonesty; but as I began to do this, I was amazed at how many times I later "saw" the blueness or realized that there are different ways of perceiving in almost any situation. This has made me feel much more comfortable with people who see things differently from the way I see them.

4. Don't Threaten Abandonment in the Face of Conflict

Threatening abandonment is something people often use to alarm their partners when they realize they're not winning. If you find your-self slipping into an argument and the partner is winning, try to avoid saying something like, "I'm going out and I don't know when I'm coming back" or "Maybe we shouldn't even be in a relationship together."

You may negotiate space, however, if you sense the discussion escalating into unbearable intensity. To do this without threatening abandonment, indicate when you will return by saying something like, "I need a time out and I'll be back to discuss this in two hours." Then keep your word and show up again in two hours.

5. Communicate in Four Sentences or Less

Here is a very helpful guideline I learned from Janet. Before making requests, describing events, or asking for support, think about what you're going to say and try to say it in four sentences and with one breath.

In addition, in your four sentences, avoid these common pitfalls:

- Try to avoid complaining.
- Try to avoid blaming, which is making one person right and the other person wrong. Complaining and blaming both make it hard for your partner to pay attention to what you're saying, even if it's reasonable.
- Try to eliminate explaining or justifying why you are doing what you are doing. Sometimes one person challenges the other and demands an explanation for that person's behavior or choices. Responding to such a challenge with justifications and explanations is not necessary. Adults don't need to

explain themselves to other adults. When you start explaining yourself, the listener often stops paying attention, realizing that a lecture or a cover-up is in the making. No one likes to be lectured, and Love Avoidants are often hypersensitive to this.

For example, before recovery Jeannie used to spend ten minutes asking her roommate Betty to get a loaf of bread at the grocery before she came home. Jeannie would talk about how poorly she slept and how her head ached as justification for not going to the store herself. Betty often didn't quite understand what Jeannie was asking for and didn't stop for bread, causing Jeannie disappointment and an argument. Now Jeannie says, "Betty, would you get some bread on your way home?" Betty replies, "Okay." And that's all they need to say about it. Of course, if circumstances have changed, or you need to change plans that involve the other person, a brief explanation is courteous.

Don't Worry About Whether Your Partner Uses These Guidelines

These guidelines are for you to follow. Whether your partner is following them or not is none of your business. If you follow them, the changes you will experience will bring you closer to being functional.

If your children say to you, "Mom, Dad is saying this about you. What's your side of the story?" you can give them some information without making him wrong. You say, "This is my perception of it." You avoid making him wrong by just explaining your perception of the matter they have asked about. And you resist going into any other matters that are not your children's concern. Stick to the subject and keep it brief.

If the other party assigns blame and calls you wrong, focus on setting a healthy internal boundary, and respond with good manners and pleasantness. Assume an attitude of observation, saying to yourself calmly, "Oh, look, my partner is assigning blame. My partner is experiencing that first core symptom, making me wrong and him (or her) right. Isn't that interesting." You just notice the person doing it without mentioning your observation. When your partner finishes, you just nod your head, evidencing the fact that you heard what was said, and go on with whatever you're doing. Besides the fact that it is a healthy way to relate, the "recovery" reason for exercising good manners is to avoid giving your partner ammunition with which to become upset about you.

INTELLECT IS THE PRIMARY TOOL FOR RECOVERY

In this observing mode, we are guided by our intellect rather than our emotions. Recovery is done primarily in the brain—we can create an intense emotional experience by what we think.

For example, your first thought may be, "I'm being victimized by these accusations that I'm wrong and she's right!" And an accompanying emotional tornado starts to form. As you do more rational, logical thinking, and hold yourself accountable for what's going on within yourself, you can do a great deal to tone down or even avoid creating a toxic emotional experience. I find it helpful to straighten out intensity-prone thinking by moving into the observing process, silently noting, "Isn't it interesting that my partner is assigning blame . . ." or arguing facts, or keeping score, or whatever the behavior is.

THE PROPER PLACE FOR
EMOTIONS IN RECOVERY

When I suggest that recovery is done primarily with the intellect, I don't mean to imply that you should become dead emotionally. A person in recovery certainly has access to mature, adult emotions, feels them, and expresses them appropriately. Recovering people don't always make decisions about how to behave based primarily on what they are feeling; and as recovery progresses they don't tap into dysfunctional, extreme emotion as often or as intensely. A good way to begin to restore a relationship is first to take care of your own emotional intensity, and then approach the relationship with some healthy control of your emotions and the behavior choices you make with regard to them. Very few relationships work well if one partner frequently vomits his or her emotions on the other.

Approaching your partner in a relationship primarily out of your intellect, refraining from reacting to your partner's inappropriate behavior, and setting strong internal boundaries assumes that you have done detoxification work about your childhood abuse. You no longer have a seething storehouse of carried or child feeling reality ready to explode and interfere, especially the feeling of shame that makes you feel worthless and often triggers anger.

As we've seen, codependents experience quite a few intense emotions about current events that are not mature adult feelings but stem from other sources. For example, a codependent may easily pick up and carry feelings for others.[1] Codependents are also prone to harbor feelings picked up during childhood from parents and to project them onto others in adult life. In addition, codependents can quickly

1See the section on carried feelings in *Facing Codependence*, by Pia Mellody with Andrea Wells Miller and J. Keith Miller (San Francisco: Harper & Row, 1"8"), 96–103.

sink into a child ego state when current events trigger a child feeling reality that was not sufficiently dealt with during childhood. When we sink into the child ego state, we feel small, vulnerable, and often defensive.

Even in recovery, however, these old feelings will continue to come up to a certain degree. The difference is that when they do come up, you can unload them with a sponsor or with friends who are mature enough to listen to them. This will prevent you from using these strong feelings from childhood to create intensity within your recovering relationship.

I've heard many people in recovery describe how they come home ahead of their partner, call a friend, and vent their anger about their partner to their friend, thus defusing their emotional intensity. Then when the partner comes home they can say, "Hi, how was your day?" in a friendly tone, and the relationship becomes much more pleasant. I recommend that recovering people discharge their leftover intense emotions with a sponsor or friend, so they can put on their boundaries and be reasonable in the presence of the partner, regardless of what the partner is doing.

Sometimes even reasonably functional people dump their emotions on one another. I just mention this to warn you to watch out for it, and to say that there is no perfection even in recovery. The point is to get more healthy and to get a better grip on yourself, to become a more responsible partner in the relationship, whether your partner is being responsible or not.

IF THERE'S NO RELATIONSHIP TO REENTER

If you are a recovering Love Addict (or Love Avoidant), it may be that you do not have a relationship to reenter. You have done the work to

detoxify old feelings related to childhood experiences of abandonment, enmeshment, or both, have done codependence recovery, and
are staying sober from any addictions. You are ready for phase four,
being in a relationship, but you have no appropriate partner. Let's say
your co-addicted relationship was a romantic-sexual one. Perhaps
your last partner has already begun another relationship, or you have
realized your former partner is not able to be supportive enough for
a healthy relationship. There are any number of reasons why you
might not have a relationship on hold to reenter.

In this situation your next step is to discover someone with whom
to socialize, and move toward forming a friendship with that person.
It's usually easier if a person is inviting you into a friendship or relationship by indicating interest in you. If there is such a person, smile
and say "yes" to a reasonable approach. If not, look for someone who
would be appropriate to ask out and begin to create a friendship—a
nonsexual social experience—with that person.

Qualifications of the New Friend

For you to benefit most from this process, this new person must not
be seriously involved with anyone else, and must be available to have
an appropriate noncompetitive relationship with you. Also it is helpful to be attracted to the person both personally and sexually. If no
such person is immediately obvious, it is helpful to your recovery to
find someone; and it is perfectly acceptable to be actively looking,
involving yourself in social experiences so you can find a person to
whom to relate.

Finding the "Perfect Person"

In our society we are urged to begin by finding someone to whom we
are physically attracted, to start a sexually intimate relationship, and
then to try to work through all the conflicts in the intellectual and
emotional areas of intimacy. I believe we need to learn how to do the

reverse: Learn to enjoy someone as an individual human being before moving into a sexually intimate relationship. But many of us think we need to find someone who fits an ideal physical image that we feel sexually attracted to before we're willing to invest anything in forming a relationship. Often it seems that there aren't many people available who qualify, and the few who do qualify don't seem to be attracted to us, especially if our own physical appearance is less than perfect.

If we can begin a friendship with someone who is pleasant or enjoyable but who may not seem physically attractive, often the less-than-perfect physical details of his or her body that first put us off become less objectionable or less important for sexual attraction. In many instances the healthy sexual attraction develops after the other areas of friendship have begun.

So if, after a while, you find no one to whom you are attracted, it may be wise to check whether you are doing something in your thinking process that makes it impossible for anyone to measure up. Some people can avoid relationships by getting out a microscope and examining every potential partner in minute detail so that almost no one can qualify. If you realize you are in this position, it might be wise to get help from a sponsor or a counselor so that you can find a way to break through your inhibiting thinking process.

Staying Nonsexual

When you have found a person—even one to whom you are physically attracted and the potential for a sexual relationship exists—I recommend that this new relationship stay nonsexual for a while, except perhaps for affectionate kissing. When I say this in a lecture, many people laugh; but I believe it is ill-advised to involve sexual drive in this process at first. You are approaching relationships from an unfamiliar and probably difficult perspective. You have learned what not to do in a relationship, but that is exactly what is most familiar to you to do. You are inexperienced at being in a relationship in a healthy way. You need all of your faculties to be alert to help you evaluate what is going on between you and the other person.

When a sexual relationship is activated, it becomes more difficult to think clearly. The drive to get closer blocks out more subtle aspects of relating and one tends to overlook vital clues about the partner's behavior. This makes it harder to track what happens in the other areas, such as intellectual, emotional, and other forms of physical and behavioral compatibility. Of course there is usually a certain level of sexual energy between the two of you, but it needs to be restrained while you begin exploring the other kinds of intimacy first.

Exploring Other Forms of Intimacy

You can practice asking for intimacy and support intellectually, emotionally, and physically, and practice responding to requests from this person. It may be that the friendship does not work out because you notice that this person can't or won't respond to your requests, or you find his or her requests difficult or inappropriate. If so, leave it and initiate another relationship. It may be difficult for a recovering Love Addict to make such a decision, but it can be a great step forward in recovery and feelings of self-worth.

Being Attracted to and Attractive to Functional People

Believe it or not, there are many functional people in our society. We haven't seen them because while we were busy in our co-addicted relationships, they didn't want to relate to us. They viewed us and all the chaos and intensity we created as difficult to be with. One of the painful aspects of recovery is becoming aware of this.

Another reason we may not have noticed many functional people is because when we were operating out of the characteristics of either a Love Addict or a Love Avoidant, we had eyes only for others like ourselves. Functional people just did not seem attractive.

Another part of recovery, then, is to change your criteria for what you find attractive. Many of the criteria will have already changed because of the maturity gained through codependence recovery.

Also, as our recovery progresses, we may become aware that the friends we have had are rather sick themselves. It's important to try to avoid judging them, and to understand that not too long ago we were a lot like they are. Also, the fact that these people are sick is none of our business. Our job is to determine the cost to us and our recovery of being around them, and to perhaps minimize contact if they will jeopardize our recovery.

These are some of the losses we may face as we become more functional. Today I notice I have great difficulty being around certain people who have this disease when it is at an intense level.

A HEALTHY RELATIONSHIP

Our childhood role models for how to carry out a relationship have proven to be inadequate. Now we are recovering from the effects of our co-addicted relationships. We are ready to try our wings, make a fresh start, and find a healthy relationship. At this point we know a lot about what not to do and relatively little about what to do. In Part III we will explore the characteristics of healthy relationships.

Part III

A Healthy Relationship

12.

MARKS OF A HEALTHY RELATIONSHIP

After you have detached from someone you have been addicted to and have worked on your codependence recovery, you have gained a degree of maturity you did not have before. This new maturity allows you to live your life differently. Above all, you are improving your relationship to your self through self-love, self-protection, self-identification, self-care, and self-containment.

You are also able to improve your relationships with other people. What does a healthy relationship entail? For a recovering Love Addict, this is an important question to answer. I had to learn from many sources, including friends, my mentor Janet, Pat Mellody, my own experience of trial and error, and other people in recovery.

CHARACTERISTICS OF A HEALTHY RELATIONSHIP

I have found nine characteristics that I have come to regard as important in promoting healthy relationships, whether with a spouse, parent, adult child, friend, or mentor. Let's look at each one in detail.

1. Each Partner Views the Other Realistically

Neither of you minimizes or denies who your partner is, nor hides your own reality from your partner. As Janet Hurley says, each of you shows up, pays attention, tells the truth, asks for what you need and want, and lets go of attachment to the outcome.

Each of you recognizes that the other is an imperfect human being, and learns what is realistic to expect. Each of you knows that your partner will make mistakes. When your partner acts offensively or violates your boundary system, each of you can deal with the violation without too much stress.

We all act offensively at times. We can violate external boundaries physically or sexually, and we can violate internal boundaries intellectually, emotionally, and spiritually. The internal boundary system is probably the one that gets transgressed most often. This happens, for example, when one person demands perfection from another, or yells or screams at the partner, is sarcastic, ridiculing, calls the partner names, or overcontrols him or her. Demanding perfection from a daughter, for instance, tells the daughter that she is not worthy as she is and triggers feelings of shame and inadequacy. Since no one can be perfect, demanding perfection is unreasonable and abusive.

In a healthy relationship you each can come to terms with occasional boundary violations without throwing your partner away or diminishing yourself in some way, although neither partner tolerates it as standard fare. Each of you knows your bottom line for maintaining identity and self-esteem and upholds it. (By bottom line I mean an event or behavior that you cannot tolerate; if the event or behavior happens you would rather leave the relationship than experience it.)

2. Each Partner Takes Responsibility for Personal Growth

Both of you continue to grow and to work on your own recovery, particularly regarding the five core symptoms of codependence. Neither of you expects your partner to do these things for you:

- Each of you practices esteeming yourself, especially during conflict with your partner. Neither of you demands that your partner esteem you at all times.
- Each of you is responsible for your own boundaries or self-protection, especially during conflict with your partner.
- Each of you can be a good listener because you have boundaries through which to filter the information coming in, enabling you to listen and pay attention to what is actually being said.
- Each of you is responsible for identifying and sharing your own physical, intellectual, emotional, and spiritual reality appropriately. Neither of you demands that the other guess your reality or allows your partner to determine it for you.
- Each of you takes responsibility for identifying your own needs and wants, and for knowing when, how, and with whom it is appropriate to reveal them. Although you are interdependent, each of you has other sources of support (such as sponsors, friends, and people in Twelve-Step or other support groups), to whom you can turn when your partner's response to your request for support needs to be "no."
- Each of you is responsible for learning to experience and express your reality in moderation. Neither of you expects the other person to tolerate extreme expressions of reality.

3. Each Partner Takes Responsibility for Staying in an Adult Ego State

Healthy people have mature adult emotions about current happenings, and recognize that their thinking creates corresponding feelings. As we saw in chapter 11, however, recovering codependents can occasionally experience old child feeling reality to a certain degree and sink into a child ego state. In a healthy relationship each partner takes responsibility for avoiding inappropriately acting out of that child ego state, communicating appropriately what is going on, and finding a way to return to an adult ego state without abusing anyone in the process.

Recovering people develop an ability to talk themselves back into an adult ego state, perhaps by getting into a private dialogue with the child within. If this isn't effective for you, you can get help from someone such as a sponsor, mature friend, or counselor.

If your partner is mature enough, you might turn to your partner for help. If you do this, however, you need to be aware of certain pitfalls for the relationship. Even though the event that triggered the lapse into a child ego state may have happened with your partner, your partner did not set up the original childhood trauma, the memory of which triggered the lapse; and your partner is not responsible for the childhood abuse and its effects. You need to be very clear with your partner at the outset that you are in a child ego state, perhaps by saying something like, "Right now I'm feeling little. I'm in a child ego state. I need some help here." Try to avoid abusing your partner through this kind of vulnerability by such ploys as expecting your partner to rescue you, or by accusing your partner of causing you to be in this child ego state in the first place.

4. Each Partner Can Focus on Solutions to Problems

Everybody has recurring problems that need to be solved. These problems come marching down life's road whether we like it or not. In a healthy relationship, each of you approaches problems by focusing on how to resolve the issue most efficiently. Then you each take responsibility for doing what you have agreed to do about the problem. Neither of you has to be right or wrong. When two people in a relationship begin trying to justify themselves or "be right," logic and recovery seem to take a vacation.

An embarrassing situation developed when I dented the fender of our truck. When I got home my husband walked up to the truck and said, "What happened?"

I said, "I didn't put the truck in park and it ran into the tree."

Pat said, "Oh. Well, I don't think we should get it fixed. It's not worth it."

And we stopped talking about it. We agreed to solve the problem by just letting the fender stay dented. He didn't once ask me, "What did you do that for?" or tell me I was stupid, careless, or incompetent. We had a very functional exchange. I realized that we had come a long way from the days when we could have loaded that dented truck with all the complaints we'd hidden for weeks before.

5. Each Partner Can Be Intimate with and Support the Partner a Reasonable Amount of the Time

When one of you expresses needs and wants, the other can be supportive as often as possible without sacrificing his or her own self-care and without doing the partner's work. In a functional relationship this is not a one-sided thing. One day you may be the one wanting or needing something, and the next day the roles may be reversed and your partner becomes the one being helped.

6. Each Partner Has Developed a Life of "Abundance"

To me, value, power, and abundance are interrelated. Value and power increase and decrease together in a synergistic way. As we value ourselves more, we empower ourselves. That is, our sense of competence to care for ourselves increases. As we empower ourselves, we increase our sense of value. Likewise, if we diminish our sense of power by our lack of self-care, our sense of value diminishes, and vice versa.

Here are two ways you can generate a sense of self-esteem or self-love that leads to feelings of being valuable: (1) Make choices in favor of yourself; and (2) act for self-care rather than react to punish somebody else for not taking care of you, not respecting you, or for doing harm to you. I've found that there is little to be gained from reacting to or punishing someone else. As you quit projecting your denied feelings so much, you may come to realize that the other person's action you dislike is often intended to take care of him or her and not designed to do you harm at all.

When we practice self-care and keep our sense of value and power at good levels, we seem to attract many kinds of abundance: friendship, money, peace, energy. This abundance further serves to enhance our sense of power and value.

I have a friend in his sixties who went for treatment and began to work on codependence recovery. He began to do affirmations. After five years he started a physical fitness program and continued to go to Twelve-Step meetings or to a counselor several times a week. This man's life began to blossom. His business, which is almost all personal contact work, is succeeding, and he is trying creative things that are working. He says that this abundance came from valuing and empowering himself and being open to the valuing and empowering of a Higher Power.

7. Each Partner Can Negotiate and Accept Compromise

As you experience increased levels of self-value, self-empowerment, and abundance, you can surrender the need to get your way all the time. You have enough energy, peace, and serenity so that you don't need to have things completely as you think they should be. Janet Hurley sums it up by pointing out that you are no longer operating out of scarcity but out of abundance, so compromise doesn't feel like something is being ripped away. Each of you can stand the anxiety of getting your wants or needs only partially met. And each of you can stand the experience of allowing your partner to operate within the partner's value system, as long as it is not abusive to the allowing partner.

For example, I like to keep things in order, preferably out of sight. I may even be a little extreme with it. Putting things away makes it easier for me to find them. My husband says that although he would like to have things neatly in their place, he finds that when he puts things out of sight he can't find them again when he needs them. He continues to work at learning how to keep track of things when they are put out of sight, although many of his belongings remain in full view so he can find them. There are piles on his desk at home, on the kitchen counter, on top of his dresser, and on his bathroom counter.

I can now smile when I describe this, but I did not find this comfortable or amusing for many years. In fact, I kept my self miserable. When I'd walk into the house, I'd see the piles, grind my teeth, and mutter, "I can't stand it. I've just got to put that away. I can't stand it, I've got to put that away." That thinking process led me to feel depressed and chaotic. It wasn't the piles themselves that upset me, it was what I thought when I looked at them.

One day I said to him, "This isn't working. I can't stand those piles. I need to put things away so I can find them."

He answered, "When you put things away, I can't find them. I don't know how to keep track of things when they're out of sight."

So I thought a minute, then I said, "We've got to do something about this. Would you be willing to reduce your pile if I'm willing not to put so much of it away?"

After thinking it over, Pat agreed to try, and so now the piles are a little smaller and a little more is put away. I am working harder to tolerate the piles that are still there, and he's working harder to learn to keep track of things that have been put away. We both compromised and things are better.

The important thing for my own internal serenity is that I have been able to move beyond thoughts that leave me feeling chaotic and depressed, to thoughts such as, "Oh, isn't that interesting? Look, the piles didn't get much bigger this week." And the feelings that come from that kind of thinking aren't so miserable.

As we began working out this compromise together, I stopped trying to control how big the piles were and whether he was going to put his shoes away. Pat began putting more away. We also decided to add six hundred square feet to the back of our house. One room of that addition is only to be used for his piles. And I promised him that I won't go into that room to clean. He agreed that I get to control what the living room looks like, and that he will keep the dogs off the furniture. You have no idea what these apparently small compromises have done for our relationship in seemingly unrelated ways.

8. Each Person Is Usually Able to Enjoy the Partner Despite the Differences Between Them

Each of you, by a conscious effort, can often keep a reasonable focus on the things you like about your partner, even when faced with something not so likable. Neither of you needs to manipulate, control, or otherwise force your partner into being a certain way so that the one manipulating can be comfortable. You maintain an acceptable comfort level by your own self-care activities, including changing the focus of your thinking about issues that have been frustrating in the past. I find that I can enjoy my partner's differences in direct proportion to how willing I am to take care of myself. The better you are at taking care of yourself, the more you will be able comfortably to let your partner be who he or she is.

9. Each Partner Can Communicate Simply and Directly

Each partner takes responsibility for making clear, direct statements concerning needs for intimacy and support, as described in chapter 11, and also for keeping these communications brief. One tool for achieving brevity is the four-sentence rule described in chapter 11.

UNREALISTIC EXPECTATIONS CAN LEAD TO DIFFICULTIES

Our expectations about what a healthy relationship ought to be often create problems for us when we attempt to form a new relationship or reenter a former relationship on a healthier basis.

One of the traits of dysfunctional codependent thinking is solving problems by thinking in extremes or swinging to the opposite pole. For example, if a person's telephone bill is too high for a few months, the person might decide the family cannot make any long distance calls at all to keep the phone bill down, or perhaps even have the telephone removed. Likewise, some people may realize that abandonment or enmeshment or using work, religion, or other activities to avoid intimacy were the reasons their relationships were so unsatisfactory. If they still solve problems by swinging to the opposite extreme, this black-and-white thinking can lead them to develop some expectations—that the partner should never go out alone, should quit his or her job, or quit going to church completely—that are fairly unrealistic, so that they have difficulty reentering relationships.

As you begin to enter or reenter a relationship after doing some recovery work on addictions and codependence, any skewed or unrealistic expectations or assumptions you hold about relationships can be more easily identified. One major clue that you are harboring such unrealistic expectations is that they are probably the triggering cause of difficulties you experience in a relationship. When a difficulty arises, try to see if one of your expectations is not being met, then see if the expectation is unrealistic.

My husband, Pat Mellody, has had some valuable insights about unrealistic expectations people develop when they begin to form relationships after entering recovery. People who hear him lecture seem to be helped to straighten out some of their skewed thinking about this area. It is our hope that these insights, given in the next chapter, will help you identify and sort through unrealistic expectations you hold and help you to become able to replace them with more realistic ones.

13.

UNREALISTIC EXPECTATIONS

by Pat Mellody

"Okay, I am ready to be in a relationship," said James, a man I had been sponsoring for about nine years.

I was delighted and curious, so I asked, "What is this lucky woman going to be like?"

He gave me a comprehensive list of attributes, including "nonjudgmental, always there for me, able to give me unconditional love." After a while I thought that his list began to sound like the Boy Scout oath: trustworthy, loyal, friendly, and so on. It seemed to me that what James was describing might be more applicable to a Labrador retriever, and also that such consistency and constancy were probably not available in a human being.

Sometimes I get confronted for being cynical about relationships, and perhaps I approach relationships with a little more skepticism than some other people do. But down deep I think relationships are wonderful. What may seem to be cynicism to others is perhaps my belief that what many recovering people hope for and expect from a relationship is not realistic to expect in anyone. I've noticed that when people hear a speaker describe what is possible in a relationship, they tend to assume these *possibilities* are what *will* probably happen. Some even go so far as to assert, "If my relationship doesn't include all these characteristics all of the time, it isn't healthy. So I probably ought to be out of this relationship and into another one."

The more I thought about unrealistic expectations such as James specified, the more I wanted to discover what realistic expectations for a good relationship might be. A few attitudes and expectations that come up regularly seem to set people up for disappointment and discouragement as they venture into healthier relationships. For example, a relationship doesn't have to include every possible positive attribute that is described in a lecture or book in order to qualify as a good relationship.

The Element of Risk: The Lady and the Tiger

Being in a relationship reminds me of the old story about the lady and the tiger: In a faraway kingdom there were laws against the princess consorting with commoners. But the king caught the princess having a romantic liaison with a common subject of the realm. When they were apprehended they were still lying together but were having a terrible lovers' quarrel. The man was hauled away to the tower with no chance even to say goodbye. The required penalty for any commoner who romanced the princess was death. But the princess, who loved the man, talked to her father, the king, and he agreed to allow the man to submit to a test.

The man would be placed in an arena with two doors. Behind one door was a tiger. If this door were opened, the tiger would leap out and kill him. Behind the other was the princess, and if he opened this door, he would be allowed to marry her. The princess, working through devious means, found out which door was which and sent this message to him: "Open the left-hand door." The question in his mind is, what did she tell him? Would she rather have him dead or married to her?

I think all relationships have a similar, though not quite so lethal, element of risk or surprise that keeps them interesting.

Relationships require trust. The problems come when we do not recognize that trust is not a decision, but the result of certain actions. Trust is the result of taking risks over time and not getting hurt. To someone who first enters a treatment center, the counselors seem to be speaking a foreign language, asking him or her to do really strange things, and saying, "Trust the process." I prefer a different way of putting it: "Take some risks in the process, and if you don't get hurt, you might trust it." But unrealistic expectations, not discussed, can lead to pain in taking risks, and that pain can destroy the willingness to trust in the future.

UNREALISTIC EXPECTATIONS

Following are several unrealistic expectations about aspects of a healthy relationship. I'd like to address them, and then suggest a more realistic approach.

1. I Will Find My Perfect Partner When I Achieve Enough Recovery

It is so easy for many of us to come to expect perfection from ourselves, our spouses, and our relationships. Sometimes we think that when we have been in recovery long enough, we will eventually achieve perfection and then will have the ability to recognize and attract the Perfect Partner. I've often told aftercare groups I've led that nothing in a relationship is improved by the fact of marriage. The marriage ceremony is about commitment to a relationship.

Improving the quality of a relationship involves some of the recovery processes that have been discussed in this book.

To compound this difficulty, many people don't define any specific goals for their recovery. All they say is "I want to be recovered" or "I am in recovery" without finding out how recovery looks in concrete terms. So we either have a clear picture of a perfect partner, as James did, or we have only a vague picture of how we will be and what our relationships will be like when we are recovered; and we just kind of wander toward these things. But underlying this wandering is the assumption that at some point in the future we will achieve Complete Recovery and enjoy Perfect Relationships.

When our wandering brings us close to the vague picture of recovery, we readjust the picture and move it further away—like a mirage moving across the desert ahead of us. At any moment we can compare where we are to where we think we ought to be, and come up short. I can see myself as being a failure in my life, my relationships, or my work simply because I am not "where I am supposed to be."

A SUGGESTED REALISTIC EXPECTATION

Both in our relationships and in the rest of our lives, we need to look at what we can realistically expect. We need to understand that we do not have a vast pool of people with perfect characteristics waiting for us out there. No matter what relationship we get into, some aspects of it will be positive and some negative. Not to realize this is to set ourselves and our prospective partners up for certain pain and disappointment.

To avoid the unrealistic expectation of either perfect recovery or perfect relationships, we need to step back and look at where we were last year, last month, or even last week. Recovery is about improvement, not perfection.

A major step for me was understanding that in recovery the journey is the goal. The journey involves being moderately comfortable on a daily basis, doing what I can about recovery today, being honest, and treating others fairly as much as I can. Following this path leads to progress and growth. Big new successes may or may not happen; but unless we learn to live sanely one day at a time, we will most likely sabotage any outstanding breaks or relationship opportunities that come along.

The program slogan about living one day at a time applies to this concept. Sometimes people use this slogan as an excuse to avoid responsibility. For example, one might think, "Since I don't have to pay the rent today, I don't need to take care of my money." But at the end of the month, when there is no money for rent, the landlord may feel differently about it. To me "One Day at a Time" is an obligation to do what I can today to insure my recovery and my future and to take care of my family. But by the same token, it means not to beat myself up if I can't get everything done today and not to keep score about whether I am "where I ought to be." Just as many of us recovering people have grandiose ideas about what other people should be like, we often have grossly inflated and unrealistic notions about how much we can accomplish in a day. We must learn how to correct these expectations, or we may dump them on our partners as well as keep ourselves in misery and in a swamp of unnecessary and unrealistic perceptions of failure.

Pia has pointed out that our recovery is done mostly with our minds, rather than following where our emotions lead us. I agree that while it is important to be in touch with our emotions, we need to recognize that healthy decisions are made at a rational level. We take input from our emotions and from other data, but it is with the intellect that we need to make decisions. Making decisions for living based primarily or entirely on what we feel like doing usually leads away from recovery.

2. If a Relationship Ends, It Was a Failure

A recovering friend who had just ended a romantic relationship said to me one day, "You know, it's not the breaking up that hurts so much as it is having another failure."

I asked, "What makes you say it was a failure?"

He said, "Well, we are not together anymore."

As I reflected on this tendency to label relationships that end as failures, I saw that believing a relationship that ends was a failure automatically makes dating a higher-risk venture than it needs to be.

And then I remembered several previous relationships of my own about which I could now feel successful because I was no longer in them. Let's say two people start a relationship and begin to negotiate life together. After they've learned more about each other, one or both of them decide that a lifetime commitment to this relationship is not a good idea, so they break up and don't get married. I consider their experience together quite successful. They entered into the process; they experimented with it; they learned things about how they operate in a relationship and what they can tolerate; they discovered it wasn't in their mutual best interest to continue pursuing the relationship; and they stopped.

A SUGGESTED REALISTIC EXPECTATION

A more realistic way to regard broken relationships might be to consider the relationship as a learning laboratory, whether the relationship eventually ends or it becomes a lifetime commitment. The pain associated with believing that the end of a relationship is a failure can thereby be greatly reduced.

3. In Healthy Relationships People Solve Problems by Discussing Them Rationally and Reasonably

It seems to be a popular misconception that after enough time has passed, two people will know each other well enough that arguments are not necessary. But I don't think it is possible to have a relationship in which people don't have disagreements, fights, or arguments, each occasionally continuing to misunderstand what the other says or does.

It seems to me that the pattern many arguments often follow is roughly like this: One partner says something that offends the other. They talk about the issue for about two sentences, and then the issue that started the argument is forgotten. Now irrationality sets in, and the partners move into trying to hurt each other emotionally and put each other down in an effort to "win" the argument or "be right." Eventually one person may say something about the issue that is fairly rational and objective, and that is not blaming, and the irrational energy can begin to dissipate. Then the two parties may get back to a productive discussion of the issue again.

A SUGGESTED REALISTIC EXPECTATION

Occasional arguments, disagreements, and even nonphysical fights are ways to practice setting boundaries and negotiate differences. It is realistic to make allowances for the irrational, emotional parts by recognizing that the irrational emotional factors in disagreements and arguments often come from a variety of personal quirks that we bring with us into a relationship. For example, I find that my getting upset and irrational during an argument has to do with my thinking I am "not being heard." When I think someone is misinterpreting what I am saying, then I start thinking the person is doing so deliberately, and I want that person to change and think like I do.

And my anger about that may supersede the anger about the original subject of the argument.

I believe this must go back to my childhood issues, because my intensity level is far bigger than the subject usually warrants. This is a painful obstacle to my ability to relate. And after many years in recovery, although I have become more aware and have gotten a little better, it doesn't look like this impulsive way of thinking is going to improve much more, as much as I wish it might. I recognize that when I am in an argument this fear of being misunderstood and discounted is likely to occur. But now when it happens I can sometimes just say, "There I go again," make amends, and get back on track. So with this realistic awareness and attitude, I don't think this obstacle is something over which I have to end a lot of relationships.

Instead of being disappointed that there is an argument, or that during it one or both people became irrational for a while, it is realistic to concentrate on seeing it through to resolution, since the disagreements are going to happen anyway. As long as the hurting phase is not beyond one's tolerance level, such as a physical fight or extreme emotional abuse, to walk out during the irrational, painful part of an argument is to risk staying in that unresolved state indefinitely. One danger is that the partner walking away may repress the issue and "get back at" the other person in passive/aggressive ways, often regarding other issues that are not apparently connected to the original, repressed argument.

4. We Will Have No Conflict Over Maintaining Mutually Desired Codes of Behavior and Characteristics of the Relationship

Two people may have similar ideas about the codes of behavior and characteristics they want in their relationship. It is unrealistic, however, to think that their understanding of these codes of behavior and characteristics will be alike. Most people have different interpretations of different characteristics, and a person's own interpretations may vary from time to time. I define the terms of the relationship from within my value system, and you define them from within yours.

Let's look at the different ways partners have of viewing a few highly prized attributes: availability, fun, unconditional love, and sexual fidelity.

First let's think about what availability means. To you, being available might mean that the other party always make room for you whenever you need her or him. But underlying this is the expectation that each would somehow know when a need was a priority to the other person.

Can we expect this kind of mind-reading? Sometimes I know which of someone's needs are a priority for that person, and sometimes I don't. Our own needs fluctuate as well. On some days, for example, I wish Pia had an on/off switch and I could keep her in the front closet. I could then wheel her out of the closet, turn the switch to "on," and say "Relationship." And when I was ready to do something else, I could turn the switch to "off" and put her back in the closet. By this method she would always be available when I wanted her, and I wouldn't have to consider any of her needs, wants, or priorities.

"Fun" is another example of a term that is rarely defined the same way by everyone. If what I think is fun happens to be near what Pia thinks is fun, we can share that. But many times, it isn't.

For instance, Pia has fun shopping. I would rather go to the dentist than shop—unless it's in a hardware store, where I have fun. There are many activities that we don't agree are fun. So most of the time we leave each other space to enjoy the fun things we each like that the other doesn't like, and only try to do things together that we both like. Among those we enjoy together are flying, gardening, and developing new lectures and treatment concepts.

Another attribute that is difficult to define is unconditional love. Most of us believe that we give but do not receive unconditional love, and we conclude that we are not loved if we perceive someone's regard for us isn't unconditional—the way we define it.

One definition I often hear is that unconditional love means a person loves another for who that person is, no matter what. Another definition might be that a person always likes everything the other does and never gets angry with that person. Again the problem is that two people's definitions of unconditional love may not be the same.

Many times what we call love is actually lust, or sexual attraction, or passion. We often call having sex making love. But having sex is just having sex. Sex can occur between two people in a loving relationship, or not. Sex can be nurturing if it is part of a loving relationship. Sometimes sex is wonderful, and sometimes it is just aerobic exercise and doesn't necessarily have anything to do with love at all.

However, sexual fidelity, the next attribute in this discussion, is a different matter. This term has many layers of meaning that present opportunities for differing definitions. On one level, fidelity might be defined as refraining from having sex with anyone but one's primary partner; on another level, fidelity is not only refraining from having sex with anyone else, but also refraining from investing emotional energy in a relationship with anyone else.

But let's assume that both people in a romantic-sexual relationship agree that fidelity refers to sexual intimacy only. On the next level, the question is, how does each person define sexual fidelity exactly? Perhaps it could be defined as not engaging in unacceptable sexual behavior outside the relationship. But what does that mean in specific and practical terms?

I believe each of us, somewhere in our subconscious minds, has a picture of what arouses us sexually. When someone who fits the picture walks by, we have a sexual response. So let's say I'm out and someone who fits my idea of a sexually attractive female walks by. From that point on, what behavior is unacceptable? Does unacceptable sexual behavior mean intercourse, or lusting after someone, or flirting, or what?

I define unacceptable sexual activity as acting in a way that is outside of one's value system. In my value system, physical sexual fidelity is essential. And that includes not engaging in sexual intercourse or physical activities designed to arouse one toward sexual intercourse. But that may or may not be how someone else would see it.

In an ideal world, infidelity would mean doing something outside of what two people have agreed on as fidelity. But how many people discuss this important definition with their partner until they settle on a meaning that they both could live by? Most marriage vows include a statement that the two people promise to be faithful, but there is no definition of what faithful means. The vast majority of couples have never intentionally agreed on what behaviors are and are not "faithful." Since a husband's value system about fidelity may be different than a wife's, there can be a lot of conflict over that issue.

A SUGGESTED REALISTIC EXPECTATION

I strongly believe that both people in a relationship need to discuss the way they understand the codes of behavior and characteristics they both want to respect in their relationship. Such discussions about what these terms mean to each person is vital, in my opinion, for deciding whether to enter a relationship with someone or not. We can hardly realistically expect to have our partner just happen to have the same understanding of what all these codes and characteristics mean.

It is my guess that very few couples contemplating marriage have sat down together and made up an exhaustive list of codes of behavior and characteristics that each expects from the partner and from the relationship and negotiated each one of them. Usually we married someone first, then we negotiated compromises—overtly or covertly.

Misunderstandings, especially about the meaning of sexual fidelity, have led to so much difficulty in so many relationships I know of, that I believe it is very important for each couple to discuss this particular issue especially as a part of their preparation for marriage. As a matter of fact, I believe that agreeing on the meaning of sexual fidelity is essential for a healthy decision regarding whether or not to enter a relationship.

5. Intimacy Will Be Natural and Easy

Another much prized but unrealistic expectation characteristic on the list is that intimacy will be natural and easy. One definition of intimacy is the act of sharing with someone exactly who you are in the moment. Another definition of intimacy, which I heard Masters and Johnson propose during a lecture on television, is sharing in each other's vulnerability. As we have seen, there are several kinds of intimacy, including physical, sexual, intellectual, emotional, and spiritual.

As Pia has established so well, intimacy in a close relationship requires healthy boundaries, self-esteem from within each person, being in touch with who we are, and knowing when it is appropriate to reveal who we are to someone and when it isn't. It is also necessary that people with whom we share are trustworthy.

A SUGGESTED REALISTIC EXPECTATION

Healthy intimacy in a close relationship is difficult. It requires work, commitment, stamina, and the willingness to risk. It is not always automatically easy, no matter how close the relationship. When we revert to childhood fears, for instance, intimacy may suddenly be practically impossible.

Also, it is sometimes harder for me to be vulnerable with someone close to me than it is to be vulnerable with a stranger, because a stranger doesn't have much power in my life. So sometimes I can sit on an airplane with a man I have never seen before and discuss many personal details about my life, even perhaps some of my fears. But in a close relationship I run a risk: If I expose these vulnerable things, the next time we fight my partner may use that personal information as a painful weapon to hurt me. And I know I'm just as likely to do that to my partner.

The fear of being hurt by someone using personal information against us is very substantial. This is true because many of us have been hurt in relationships with people with whom it was unsafe to share, and we have been unsafe ourselves. Only after much recovery do we begin to learn to fight fairly and to become a person who deserves to be trusted with vulnerable information. So, while it would be nice to feel safe enough to have deep intimacy, it is actually often a risk. Even so, as I continue in recovery, improve my boundaries, and seek out people in recovery with whom it is safe to share, I am willing to risk more often. Happily I find that I do experience such intimacy more and more often, and therefore I am beginning to develop some trust. It has been important to me to realize that my trust doesn't have to be only in the person with whom I am sharing. I can now sometimes trust my boundaries, my self-esteem, the recovery process, and my Higher Power.

6. All Our Needs Will Be Met All the Time

My search for what is realistic to expect from a relationship includes considering the various needs and wants that could possibly be met in a relationship. The list of possibilities is endless. For example, here is a list of things people usually suggest when I ask, "What are some of the more desirable characteristics of a good relationship?"

Ability to compromise	Intimacy
Accommodation	Loyalty

Affirmation

Love, passion

Availability

Negotiation

Common interests

Openness

Communication

A partner

Companionship

Reliability

Confrontation

Respect for boundaries

Fidelity

Sex

Fun

Trust

Good cooking

Willingness

Honesty

A SUGGESTED REALISTIC EXPECTATION

I think that the most important ingredient in a comfortable relationship (and it takes a lot of recovery) is acceptance. And part of what I accept is that I don't have all these characteristics in my partner, in the relationship, or in myself. Some I have most of the time, some I don't have at all. The characteristics I do have come and go depending on my levels of recovery, sensitivity, and awareness of my own reality each day.

Recovery, in my opinion, deals directly with finding a mature way to be honest and moderately comfortable on a daily basis. As codependents we usually want even our recovery to be extreme. If we've had a lot of pain, seriousness, and conflict, we want recovery to be full of joy, fun, and harmony all the time. But real life includes experiences ranging from extreme pain to absolute joy, and most of the time it hovers around the middle range of those limits. There is a dividing line somewhere between each end of the spectrum that separates comfort-to-joy from discomfort-to-pain. Our experience in a good relationship fluctuates up and down along this spectrum. If our experience in a relationship can be on the comfort side of the dividing line most of the time, I think we are doing pretty well.

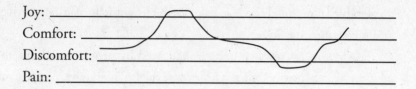

We also need to accept the fact that we get below the comfort line some of the time not because we are recovering addicts, but because that is the way life is for everyone. I am now moderately comfortable on a daily basis. That is so much better than it used to be, when my feelings ranged from uncomfortable to terrible pain and thoughts of suicide. At one time I believed joy was the absence of pain. It is only in recent years that I have realized that joy and pain can coexist in a healthy person, and that I have begun to be aware of the full spectrum of experiences in my relationships and be satisfied that things are still going well.

7. Problems Mean I Need to End My Relationship

When people enter a new relationship and then encounter problems, many often think that ending the relationship is the best or only solution. When problems are large enough or stubborn enough, sometimes they indicate that a relationship does need to end. But I think we need to refrain from jumping to that conclusion too hastily, without considering a few things—such as the number of satisfying areas about the relationship and whether or not the problems can be negotiated.

A SUGGESTED REALISTIC EXPECTATION

Many people who are in a relationship and encounter some negative aspects need to it ask themselves whether their relationship is something they really want to attempt. But even as we consider getting out of a relationship, I think we need to look at which needs are being met versus which ones aren't. How much of the relationship is intolerable, how much of it is tolerable? How much of it is positive and how much negative?

Satisfied needs tend to be overshadowed by problems. Abraham Maslow was a psychologist who established a hierarchy of human needs, ranging from the most basic to higher levels of human experience. He pointed out that when we have more than one need at once, the most basic one seems the most pressing until it is satisfied, then the next one becomes pressing. He also said, "A satisfied need is not a motivator." In other words, we are not motivated to act by needs that are satisfied. In fact, we humans have difficulty keeping in touch with a need once it is being met. We often say we don't have a need for something, when in actuality we still have the need, but it is satisfied for the moment.

Here's an illustration. Let's say that a soldier parachutes to the wrong place and is lost in the desert. He wanders around with no provisions for about a day or so, and then he's rescued. The first thing he needs right away is water. Water is often considered the most basic physical need. When we need water we notice it and say, "Boy, am I thirsty," then drink some water. But I cannot recall ever hearing anyone say, "You know, I'm not thirsty. I haven't been thirsty all day. When I was a younger man I used to be thirsty all the time, but nowadays I am just not thirsty like I used to be."

After drinking some water, the next needs our soldier would notice would be for food and then rest. Instead of spending the rest of the day thinking how he is not thirsty anymore, the soldier starts thinking about how hungry he is, and then how tired he is. He no longer consciously identifies the needs that are being met.

This concept is extremely important in relationships. When we feel the aggravation of our unmet needs, we usually don't take stock of all our needs that have been met.

As an example of how this could affect a relationship, let's take a look at the life of a man I'll call Sam. Years ago Sam, the manager of a large store, was married to his first wife. They had two children and lived in a three-bedroom house. There were many good things in that relationship. Sam had a boat and membership in a shooting club, among other things. He liked old guns and had two or three. He and his wife had mutual friends, mutual respect. But Sam didn't think that his sex life was adequate. He focused on that, and as a result he left his wife and kids.

Sam believed if he could just get a really loving, sexual relationship, everything would be great. Eventually he met someone and had a really loving, sexual partner. But then Sam came very close to suicide—because once that need was met, the sexual relationship became relatively unimportant. While sex was there when he wanted it, many of the other things that were very important to him were gone. He no longer had his children, he didn't have as many mutual interests, or as much mutual respect, with his new wife. He didn't have the material things he had had before, such as his boat and his membership in a shooting club. Sam's guns were all stored in the basement and he had no place to shoot.

To satisfy one or two needs, Sam let go of all the rest and ended up living in a small efficiency apartment without many of the things that made him comfortable.

Sam's experience taught me something really important: So many times we do not look at the needs that are being met, or count our blessings. To count our blessings is to examine on a fairly regular basis in some sort of practical way what needs we have that are being met.

EVALUATING A RELATIONSHIP

When we start thinking about whether to get out of a relationship, I suggest that we take several steps.

First, we look at the problems in the relationship. Next, we determine our tolerance level. There is usually a level below which what goes on in the relationship is intolerable, and above which what goes on is tolerable. We need to determine whether these problems are above or below our comfort line. Since many of us were not taught how to meet or evaluate our needs and wants as children (core symptom four of codependence), we may well need some help from a counselor to evaluate and answer these questions.

Is there enough safety in the relationship physically, sexually, intellectually, spiritually, and emotionally? Am I getting assaulted in any of these areas? I don't think it is wise to stay in a physically violent relationship. The violence can escalate very quickly, and steps must be taken at the first signs of physical violence to assure the physical safety of the other family members.

On the other hand, whether to stay in an emotionally abusive relationship is a judgment call. I think it depends on how emotionally abusive the partner is and how good one's boundaries are. There is a wide spectrum of emotional abuse. For example, our partner might stand close to us (violating our physical boundary) and scream at us or ridicule us with cruel sarcasm (violating our emotional boundaries) on a daily basis. This is at the extremely abusive end of the spectrum, and is in some ways worse than physical abuse. But toward the less extreme end of the spectrum, our partner might make snide comments about our cooking in a normal tone of voice, while standing an acceptable distance away. We may be able to tolerate this level of intensity if we have strong boundaries and a strong sense of self-esteem. Each of us needs to get what help we need to see past our denial and determine our own individual tolerance levels.

Next, I believe it is helpful to review all the things in the relationship that are satisfactory or even enjoyable. For example, a couple may feel very compatible about how they raise the kids together, or about how they deal with financial matters. They may feel great satisfaction with their social life, or they may be supportive of each other's work.

During the evaluation period, each person develops a list of what is positive or above the comfort line, along with what is below the comfort line.

After these steps have been taken, each person can begin to negotiate the issues that are less than tolerable but close to the comfort line. Each person asks the other, "Can we start working on these? Are they negotiable?"

Then, after evaluating the problems and attempting to negotiate the areas that have been deemed less than tolerable, each person has more data with which to determine whether to stay in a relationship or not.

DEVELOPING AND MAINTAINING
REALISTIC EXPECTATIONS

To get and keep realistic expectations about relationships, many of us need to adjust the way we look at some things. We need to learn or relearn how to reasonably approach relating to others. We can begin by learning not to be so critical of ourselves and others. It is helpful to get periodic feedback from a sponsor, a counselor, or someone else in recovery who can not only confront our skewed and critical thinking and behavior, but can also confront us when we want to beat ourselves up so much that we cannot look at how our relationships and lives have improved.

Much of relating to someone is evidently a matter of accepting that there are some areas on which we and our partners will never agree. I have discovered that there are some subjects Pia and I had best not talk about, because we have decided that even after knowing each other now for a long time, our discussion of these subjects is likely to lead us into a fight. And since the issues are not below our tolerance levels, we can detach and agree to disagree. The good things about our relationship outweigh the discomfort of disagreeing on particular issues.

In recovery we need to learn or relearn acceptance of ourselves, the impact of our addictions and of codependence on our lives and our relationships, and the necessity for continuing the recovery process. Along with this self-acceptance we need to develop and maintain realistic expectations for our recovery and relationships and the acceptance of things we cannot change. These, I believe, constitute the cornerstone on which healthy relationships can be built.

Part IV

JOURNALING EXERCISES
FOR RECOVERY

14.

JOURNALING EXERCISES
FOR FACING
LOVE ADDICTION

In this chapter we will look at how love addiction may have operated in your life, and what you can begin to do to recover. We will assume that you realize that you are in, or have been in, a co-addicted relationship, and that you want to recover.

First, we will explore how you have experienced both the symptoms of love addiction and the stages in the cycle of love addiction. By doing this you can begin to accomplish the first two steps in addiction recovery: to come more fully out of denial about the addiction, and to examine the harmful consequences of being in this addiction. Then, as you intervene on the addictive process of your co-addicted relationship, the journaling exercises will help you see how you experience the symptoms of codependence and how you can begin to improve in those areas.

The more relationships in your adult life that you can identify as having love addiction characteristics, the more you can confront your addiction. Write about each person with whom you've had a co-addicted relationship, whether the relationship is still existing or not.

Not all relationships are necessarily love addicted. Some people form addictive relationships only with romantic relationships, while others may have a co-addicted relationship only with a parent or child, or with a close friend, minister, or counselor.

THE SYMPTOMS OF LOVE ADDICTION

Describe how you have experienced each of the three major symptoms of Love Addiction as listed below, and the harmful consequences of each instance described. Do this exercise for each person to whom you have been addicted.

1. A disproportionate amount of time, attention, and value above myself.
2. Expectation of unconditional positive regard at all times.
3. Self-care activities I neglected because of my focus on my partner in our co-addicted relationship.

Example
    Name of Person: *Mother*
    Type of Relationship: *Parent*
    Duration of Relationship: All my life
    1. Too much time, attention, and value above myself:

Time spent obsessing about this person. (Too much time and attention.)	How I made this person my Higher Power. (Assigned value above myself.)	Harmful consequences
I sat at work thinking for two hours about my last telephone talk with my mother, obsessing about what I could say to make her understand me and see my point of view.		I was thirty minutes late for a conference with my boss and got in trouble. I haven't finished a report due yesterday about a new project.
	Mother said that having my résumé done by a professional company was expensive and not that much better than I could do myself. Even though she's never worked, done a résumé, or seen one, I decided not to hire the professionals and to do the résumé myself. I lost the job I wanted.	The woman who got the job had qualifications similar to mine. Her professional résumé presented her qualifications better than my amateur résumé had.

(Other examples of harmful consequences are described in chapter 9.)

Example

2. Expectation of unconditional positive regard at all times.

Description of my behavior	Harmful impact on other person	Response I expected	Actual response of other person
I agreed to meet my boyfriend for lunch at noon, but was late. When he was angry, I cried and told him he didn't love me or else he wouldn't be angry.	He had rushed away from the office and had to sit in the waiting area of the restaurant. My being late made him late to an important meeting. He felt pain and anger about my saying he didn't love me because he had a normal response to my being late.	I expected him to overlook the inconvenience of having to wait and to be glad to see me. I thought when you love someone you never get angry at him or her.	He was angry that he rushed away from his office only to have to wait, and also that he would now be late to his afternoon meeting.

Example

3. Self-care activities I either don't do for myself or have discontinued doing for myself that I believe this person does for me, or that I believe this person should do for me (whether the person actually does them or not).

Description of how I act needy and neglect myself	What this person does to take care of me in this area and/or how I manipulate him or her to do so
I don't eat properly and pretend I don't know how to do so.	My mother does all the cooking for me, and makes a scene if I skip meals. She packs a lunch for me to take to work.
I don't take my heart medicine, then get short of breath as a result.	My mother gets worried, watches the time, and calls me to ask if I took my pill or not.

Use the blank forms on the following pages to journal about how these characteristics operate in your own life. Write about all three characteristics for one person, then move on to write about each person to whom you have been addicted. (Feel free to copy this form in a spiral notebook.)

Name of Person:

Type of Relationship:

Duration of Relationship:

1. Too much time, attention, and value above myself.

Time spent obsessing about this person. (Too much time and attention.)	How I made this person my Higher Power. (Assigned value above myself.)	Harmful consequence

2. Expectation of unconditional positive regard at all times.

Description of my behavior	Harmful impact on other person	Response I expected	Actual response of other person

3. Self-care activities I either don't do for myself or have discontinued doing for myself that I believe this person does for me, or that I believe this person should do for me (whether the person actually does them or not).

What the person does to take care of me in this area and/or how I manipulate this person to do so	
Description of how I act needy and neglect myself	

STAGES OF THE LOVE ADDICTION CYCLE

Describe how you have experienced passing through each stage of the emotional cycle of the Love Addict. Do this for each person to whom you have been addicted.

Name of Person:
Type of Relationship:[1]
Duration of Relationship:

1. Attraction to power and seductiveness and apparant "power" of the Love Avoidant. (*Special Note:* Skip part 1 if you are writing about a son or daughter.) (Review chapter 3 for examples.)

A. How I first met this person (what happened):

B. Examples of the person's characteristics that first attracted me (power and seductiveness):

---

[1] If the person you're writing about is your son or daughter, the fantasy and breaking through denial in these emotional cycles are a little different. Look at the "Special Note" in each set of instructions to see how to write about this kind of relationship.

2. Feeling high as my fantasy was triggered:

A. How I created a fantasy in childhood about who this per
son was supposed to be in order for me to be comfortable.
Here is what I thought the "perfect" spouse, parent,
friend (whichever type of relationship this is about) would
be like. (*Special Note:* If this is about a relationship with a
son or daughter, here is my fantasy about the characteristics that this child is "supposed to" have to make me
comfortable or satisfied as a "competent" parent):

B. How I placed the face of my fantasy-partner over this person's face as our relationship developed, and refused to see
who he/she actually was (denial of person's reality):

3. Feeling relief from emotional pain of loneliness, emptiness,
and not mattering to partner.

How I began to feel valued, full, and complete because of
the experience of connecting with the Love Avoidant.

4. Showing more neediness and denying of reality of the Avoidant's walls:

> How the reality of this person's not being there for me kept coming up and I ignored what was happening. (*Special Note:* If this is about a relationship with a son or daughter, that person is not supposed to be there for me. As the parent, I am supposed to be there for the child, and release that child to his or her own life as an adult. The following is my description of how my child did not fit my predetermined idea of who he or she was supposed to be, how this discrepancy kept coming up, and how I ignored what was happening and tried to change the child to fit my preconceptions.)

5. Developing of awareness of partner's walls and behavior outside the relationship and denial crumbles:

> The event or events that broke through my fantasy about who the person is supposed to be, or my denial about being avoided. (*Special Note:* If this is about a relationship with a son or daughter, the event that breaks through this fantasy might be the child getting arrested for shoplifting or drunk driving or getting pregnant as a teenager or while not in a long-term, committed relationship.)

6. The withdrawal experience:

My emotional withdrawal experiences when my denial cracked open or my partner left:

Pain (describe)

Fear (describe)

Anger/Jealousy (describe)

7. The obsessive/planning stage:

Here are the obsessive thoughts I've had and the plans I
made regarding my partner after I came out of denial about
his or her real behavior in our relationship:

A. Here are the plans I made to relieve the emotional pain
(for example, plans to get drunk, overeat, or engage in any
addictive or compulsive action):

B. Here are the plans I made about ways to create discomfort, punish, or get even with my partner:

C. Here are the plans I made to get the relationship with the
person going again:

8. The compulsive behavior to carry out plan stage:

Date	How I carried out the above plans	Results (choose any that apply: relieved symptoms, got even, or got relationship back)

RECOVERY WORK

Now that you have faced the facts about your involvement in Love Addiction, the next step in addiction recovery is to intervene on the addiction. It is wise to move immediately into serious work on the core symptoms of codependence as you do this. Working on these symptoms will help you endure the withdrawal experience until you have time to get over the worst of its effects.

1. Describe the things you must do to stop the primary addictive processes you can identify. (Examples include: Stop chasing somebody who doesn't want to be with you. Stop having sex with inappropriate people. Stop drinking.)

2. Examine your experience with the core symptoms of codependence, especially the symptoms regarding self-esteem, acknowledging reality, and acknowledging and meeting your own needs and wants.

   A. Write about shaming experiences in childhood that affected your sense of inherent worth:

B. List any self-talk that describes you as worth less or one-
down; then write new statements that describe you
neither as one-down nor one-up:

How I would describe myself as having equal value to this person (I am neither one-down nor one-up)	
How I describe myself as being worth less than this person (I am in a one-down position)	

C. List any self-talk that describes the other person in a
   one-up position; then write new statements that describe
   this person neither as one-up nor one-down.

How I describe the other person as worth more than myself (I am in a one-down position)	How I would describe this person as having equal value as myself (I am neither one-down or one-up)

D. Describe value conflicts between you and the other
person. (Examples might include conflicts over handling
money, raising children, what to wear on various
occasions, who should do various household chores, and
so on.)

E. In your current relationship note every day the amount of time spent thinking about this person and write it down. Describe what you are thinking, then describe the reality about the person that is different from your thinking about him or her.

Date	Amount or time	What I am thinking about this person	Reality about person that is different from my thinking

F. Describe ways you neglect yourself around things you need and want. Use this information to write healthy statements about who you are and what you need and want to do for yourself.

Who I am and what I need and want to do for myself	How I neglect needs and wants

15.

WRITING A STEP ONE
FOR LOVE ADDICTION

Step One: We admitted we were powerless over_____ (name of person addicted to) and that our lives had become unmanageable.[1]

As Love Addicts, our *powerlessness* is demonstrated by attempts to control the reality of the person to whom we are or were addicted (for instance, attempts to make that person quit drinking or like dancing).

As Love Addicts, our *unmanageable* lives are due to harmful consequences created for ourselves and others as a result of our attempts to control the person to whom we are or were addicted.

Using these definitions of powerlessness (control attempts) and unmanageability (harmful consequences), list all of the people, past and present, to whom you have been or are presently addicted. This does not include just romantic or sexual relationships, but any person to whom you relate in an addictive manner.

1See page 11 for a review of how Step One helps to begin recovery.

Name	Type of relationship (sexual, friendship, parental, etc.)

Example 1

Name: Harry

Type of Relationship: Romantic/Sexual

Other Person's Reality	Powerlessness: *What I did to control this person*	Unmanageability: *Harmful results*
Body	Encouraged Harry to drink so he would be too sick to leave me	Harry almost died of alcoholism.
Thinking	Withheld information about myself so he would have a positive impression of me.	Harry felt betrayed when he found out I have herpes.
Feelings	Flirted outrageousely with another man in front of Harry to make him jealous.	Harry and this man got into a loud argument and Harry looked foolish in front of his boss. The man's girlfriend was hurt and angry.
Behavior	I acted helpless about getting my car fixed so he would take care of it and I could feel loved.	As a result of helping me, Harry now views me as less-than and helpless. I feel too dependent on him. Also, Harry didn't have time to get a haircut before his important business lunch

Example 2

Name: Alicia

Type of Relationship: Forty-year-old daughter

Other Person's Reality	Powerlessness: *What I did to control this person*	Unmanageability: *Harmful results*
Body	Told Alicia she should not wear her cocktail dress to the company Christmas party.	She didn't wear it, and everyone else got dressed up. She was embarrassed and blamed me.
Thinking	Reminded Alicia to send her grandmother (my mother) a birthday card.	Kept her from having her own consequences if she forgot, or the joy of giving from her own choice.
Feelings	Told Alicia she didn't love me because she hadn't called in weeks.	Alicia felt angry and shamed. We had an argument and shouted at each other.
Behavior	So that I could feel love, I exaggerated my heartburn so Alicia would think it was a heart attack and be afraid I might die.	Alicia sees me as incapable and less-than. She thinks I exaggerate and doesn't trust me now.

Example 3
Name: Wanda
Type of Relationship: Best friend

Other Person's Reality	Powerlessness: *What I did to control this person*	Unmanageability: *Harmful results*
Body	Told Wanda she's too old to wear her hair so long.	Wanda got angry and told me I didn't know much about attractiveness.
Thinking	Lied, telling Wanda I had a graduate degree from Stanford so she would be impressed.	Wanda felt betrayed when she bragged about my degree to a mutual friend, who told her the truth.
Feelings	Told Wanda I'd seen my husband having a drink with another woman so she'd feel sorry for me. Left out that the woman was a business client.	Wanda argued with her husband, who works with my husband. When her husband told her who the woman was, Wanda felt betrayed. My husband was hurt when he heard about what I'd said.
Behavior	Acted helpless at the last minute about baking cookies for our bridge club so Wanda would bake mine along with hers.	Wanda stayed up too late baking extra cookies and was too tired to play bridge very well. She also views me as less-than and scatterbrained.

Use the format below to describe the powerlessness and unmanageability of the relationships with people to whom you are or have been addicted. Complete a form for each person named in the list you made at the beginning of this exercise.

Name:

Type of Relationship:

Unmanageability: *Harmful results*		
Powerlessness: *What I did to control this person*		
Other Person's Reality	Body	
	Thinking	
	Feelings	
	Behavior	

16.

WRITING A STEP FOUR FOR LOVE ADDICTION

Step Four: "Made a searching and fearless moral inventory of ourselves."

A helpful way to approach writing a moral inventory about our lives as Love Addicts is to begin by examining our value system. First, we need to identify our own values. Then we can explore how we have operated outside those value systems as a result of the relationship with the person to whom we're addicted.

Loosely defined, our *value system* is the set of rules we follow about how to conduct our lives in the world so that we have integrity. When we live by these rules we feel good about ourselves. When we don't, we feel guilty and less-than.

Love addiction causes us to operate outside our value systems in several ways. When we give another person too much time, attention, and value above ourselves, we make that person our Higher Power, and consequently make that person's value system more important than our own. When we encounter a conflict between our own values and the other person's and conduct our lives according to the other person's values, we are operating outside our own value system. As we go through the cycles of emotions and hit the stage in which our denial crumbles, we see we are being abandoned, and we enter the emotional pain of withdrawal, we may resort to behaviors outside our own value system because of our obsessive and compulsive behavior. For example, we may use addictions to relieve the pain (getting drunk, or binging and purging, or going on a spending spree), with all the harmful consequences associated with them. Also, in the process of trying to get even with the Love Avoidant, we may destroy the property of others or have a sexual affair. In the process of trying to get the relationship back, we may abandon our children or other loved ones or tolerate unhealthy or injurious behavior from our partner.

The bottom line is that operating outside our own value systems creates a wide range of harmful consequences for ourselves as well as for others. We experience internal emotional anguish, guilt, and shame, and may experience other losses, including financial loss, loss of physical health, loss of employment, or loss of reputation. The harmful consequences our love addiction creates for others may include painful consequences for our children, our friends, our employer, our spouse, our parents, even total strangers (for example, we have a car wreck as a result of reckless driving while experiencing intense anger).

The following guidelines suggest several categories of life about which people have value systems. Think about your own values in each category. Then, in instances where you have operated outside your own values due to your obsession with someone to whom you were addicted, describe what you did and the harmful consequences that resulted from your behavior. Use the format on the next page for this writing.

Write about how you have operated outside of your values in any of the following categories that you feel apply to your life. This list is not intended to be a complete list of values. Add any other categories that apply especially to you:

Suggested Categories of Values

money	the way to be sexual	appropriate dress
religion	sexual fidelity	celebrating holidays
politics	having a relationship	use of leisure time
employment	parenting children	relating to parents
lifestyle	entertaining friends	social manners
food		

Example

Category of Value: Sexual fidelity

My value	How I operated outside my value	Harmful consequences
Having sex only with my wife, Pam, and no one else.	After I found out that Pam had an affair with her boss, I had an affair with Susan, whom I had met in a bar.	I feel guilty because I deceived Susan. She didn't know I was married, and was hoping I would have a relationship with her. Also, my secret affair caused me to have emotional distance from Pam. Instead of helping me get even, it made the situation worse.

Example
Category of Value: Money

My value	How I operated outside my value	Harmful consequences
Pay off credit card accounts; do not charge up to the credit limit.	My husband's value is having a good time; worrying about the money puts a damper on his fun. It's okay to charge up to the limit on credit cards and not to worry about paying them off.	I feel miserable when we go out and use the credit card. We are in tremendous debt and wasting money paying finance charges every month.

Example
Category of Value: Appropriate dress

My value	How I operated outside my value	Harmful consequences
I feel most comfortable when I'm dressed in a modest way in well-tailored, discreet clothing that covers my body well.	My husband wanted me to wear halter tops, backless sundresses, bikini bathing suits, and miniskirts. He said I shouldn't hide my body.	I feel embarrassed most of the time we go out. Other men make passes at me that I must deal with. Other women I respect are cool toward me.

Example

Category of Value: Relating to parents

My value	How I operated outside my value	Harmful consequences
I think I should visit my mother weekly in the nursing home.	My wife hates to go to the nursing home and says we pay the staff enough to look after my mother. She says my mother only whines and complains anyway, and since she has plenty of things to do there, we don't need to go. So I rarely visit her.	My mother is neglected. I feel guilty when I think about her. My sister resents my lack of attention to our mother, and our relationship is strained.

Use the blank forms on the next page to write your own moral inventory of how you have operated outside your values as the result of being in a relationship as a Love Addict. Write about every category of value you can think of that has been affected by any co-addicted relationship you have written about in the Journaling Exercises or in the Step One Exercises.

Category of Value:

My value	How I operated outside my value	Harmful consequences

17.

JOURNALING EXERCISES FOR THE LOVE AVOIDANT

This chapter provides journaling guidelines for the Love Avoidant. First, we will look at how the characteristics described in chapter 4 have operated in your relationships. Then we will look at how you have experienced the emotional cycles of a Love Avoidant in your relationships. Last we will explore what you can do to enter recovery.

CHARACTERISTICS OF THE LOVE AVOIDANT

Use the following forms to describe how you have (1) avoided intensity within your relationships by focusing on intensity outside the relationship; (2) avoided being known by the other person; and (3) avoided opportunities for intimate contact with the other person in your relationships.

Avoiding Intensity (Involvement) Within a Relationship

1. List in the left column opportunities you had for involvement with someone in a relationship, how you avoided it, and the harmful consequences for you or the other person or the relationship itself (or any combination of these).

Example

Chance for involvement with person	How I avoided involvement with this person	Harmful consequences
My daughter, Angela, won a ballet award when she was sixteen. My wife suggested I take her to New York to see a national ballet company to acknowledge her achievement.	When Angela and I got to New York, I arranged for a business associate's wife to take her to the ballet while I had a business dinner and meeting with my associate.	My daughter felt abandoned by me. I missed a chance to get to know her. I gave her the message that she isn't worth being with and that what she is good at (ballet) isn't worthwhile or interesting to me.
I made time to take my son, Frank, fishing for the first time when he was nine.	I also took a ten-year-old boy from the state foster home. I paid more attention to him than I did to Frank. When Frank acted hostile to the boy, I chewed him out in front of the other boy.	Frank felt abandoned by me. He was afraid to be mad at me, so he took it out on the boy. I shamed him by chewing him out. The boy got the brunt of Frank's feelings. Not one of us had a good time.

Use the following form to write examples from your own life:

Harmful consequences	How I avoided involvement with this person	Chance for involvement with person

2. Use the following form on the next page to describe how you created intensity outside of your important relationships and your sense of connecting to others outside your relationship.

Example

Source of intensity	Person or people involved	My sense of connection
Drinking at the Pink Elephant every Friday night.	Bartenders Tommy and Buddy, Alicia, the waitresses Sally and Kelly, regular customers Hal, Sami, Joe, Trudy, Joyce, Bobby, Nolan.	These people were like my second family. The Pink Elephant felt like my home away from home. I could relax there. I knew I was welcome.
Volunteer work to build a baseball park for the YMCA four nights a week.	Sam, John, Allison, Sandra, Jeremy, Ben.	We dedicated ourselves to something really good for the community.

Use the following form to write examples from your own life:

Source of intensity	Person or people involved	My sense of connection

Avoiding Being Known by the Other Person

1. Use the form on the next page to describe ways you have
   avoided being known by the other person in your relationship by using walls instead of healthy boundaries. Then
   describe the harmful consequences that resulted from the
   person not having the information about you. Include information about such things as a need or want, an opinion or
   preference, your feelings, or something you would like to do.

Example

Type of wall: silence, pseudo-maturity, pleasantness	How I used this wall to avoid revealing myself intimately (physical, emotional, intellectual, or behavioral)	Harmful consequences
Silence	My wife asked me if I minded if she invited her mother to visit us for Christmas. I didn't want her mother to visit because it was my family's turn to visit, but I wanted to avoid a fight.	My wife assumed I didn't mind, and invited her mother. I resented her mother's visit and wasn't very pleasant. Her mother felt uncomfortable being there.

Type of wall: silence, pseudo-maturity, pleasantness	How I used this wall to avoid revealing myself intimately (physical, emotional, intellectual, or behavioral)	Harmful consequences

2. Use the form on the next page to describe instances in which you avoided being known by dealing with something by yourself and not asking for support or help from the other person in a close relationship. This could include dealing with a problem, planning a project, or coping with emotions from a painful experience.

Example

What I dealt with alone	How I kept this to myself	Harmful consequences
Found out I had inoperable cancer.	Made the doctor promise not to tell. Told the family I had an infection. Kept all my fears and pain to myself.	My wife felt betrayed when she eventually found out. I felt lonely with my fears.
Lost my job.	Kept getting dressed and leaving the house as if going to work.	I felt lonely and afraid. My wife wound up writing bad checks without knowing I had not deposited a paycheck.

Harmful consequences	How I kept this to myself	What I dealt with alone

Avoiding Opportunities for Intimate Contact

1. Use the form on the next page to list ways you avoid opportunities for contact with your partner by such distractions as keeping the television or radio going, reading books or the newspaper, or keeping busy with projects such as home repairs, volunteer work at church or in the community, sports, and so on.

Example

Type of distraction	Describe incident in which this distraction was used	What you avoided by using this distraction
Played country and western songs very loud on the car radio.	During our last vacation, we drove from Colorado to California. I kept the radio loud enough that we couldn't talk about anything.	I avoided talking to Helen about anything. Our talks usually end up in fights, and that's not my idea of a good vacation.
Built a darkroom in the basement and spent every evening in it learning new development techniques.	My kids are noisy. My son wants help with his physics homework. He thinks because I have a degree in engineering that I'll know all the answers. My wife lurks around wanting to talk all the time.	I avoid having to help the kids with their homework. I avoid having to talk to my wife about the trouble with our marriage or the mess she made of the checkbook.

Type of distraction	Describe incident in which this distraction was used	What you avoided by using this distraction

2. Use the form on the next page to list ways you have avoided opportunities for intimate contact by controlling someone or something in the relationship.

Example

Form of control	Issue I controlled	Harmful consequences
Irritated argument	Wife's request for sex a different way than usual.	She's hurt and angry. I'm not able to perform.
Harping about spending money.	Vacation plans we make every summer.	We don't enjoy vacations for fear of overspending. Little spontaneity.
Put my son down for not being convincing in request made to me.	Son's request to stay up later.	Son doubts his thinking ability, feels shamed.

Form of control	Issue I controlled	Harmful consequences

3. As a result of being enmeshed, controlled, and used by caregivers in childhood, you may now be very sensitive to anything that might be controlling of you. Use the form on the
next page to describe things the other party does and why
you perceive him or her to be controlling. Then, in the third
column, write statements about how the other party's behavior might be to take care of himself or herself rather than to
control you.

Other person's behavior: what he or she does	How this behavior seems to be controlling	How this behavior might be the other person taking care of himself or herself
My wife asked me if I had gotten the car's inspection sticker renewed.	I'm the man of the family. I felt like a forget-ful little boy being con-trolled by a bossy mother.	My wife was about to leave alone, taking the car to visit her mother in another city, and she didn't want to be picked up by the highway patrol for not having a valid car inspection sticker.
My girlfriend asked me about my visit to my children, who live with my ex-wife.	I thought she was trying to find out about my relationship with my ex-wife.	She was initiating conversation to be verbally intimate and to see how I was doing.
My husband cleaned up the garage floor and put away all my gardening supplies so I can't find them.	He is trying to show me what a messy person I am in order to get me to clean up after myself.	My husband was cleaning out the space in the center of the garage so he could park the car there.

Use the following form to write examples from your own life:

Other person's behavior: what he or she does	How this behavior seems to be controlling	How this behavior might be the other person taking care of himself or herself

EMOTIONAL CYCLES OF THE LOVE AVOIDANT IN RELATIONSHIP WITH A LOVE ADDICT

Describe how you have experienced passing through each stage of the cycles of emotion experienced as a Love Avoidant. Do this for each person with whom you have had a co-addicted relationship. (Review chapter 5 for more examples.)

Name of Person:
Type of Relationship:
Duration of Relationship:

1. Entered the relationship out of duty and to avoid guilt:

2. "Connection" through a wall of seduction. Here is how I got our relationship going with seduction:

  A. The kinds of power I displayed that impressed this person:

  B. The ways I was attentive to this person and the needs I took care of:

  C. The ways I displayed protectiveness toward this person:

3. Feeling emotional high from adulation of the love addict. Here are the things that gave me an emotional boost at the beginning of this relationship:

4. Feeling engulfed and controlled. Here is how the neediness of the other person began to feel overwhelming:

5. Leaving the relationship. Here are the things I did to get distance from the Love Addict and our relationship (if you did):

6. Returning out of guilt or fear of abandonment or both. Here is how I decided to return to this relationship (if you did):

RECOVERY WORK

As we have seen, fear of intimacy for you, the Love Avoidant, stems from the belief that it is a draining, engulfing experience that will completely control your life. This comes from childhood experiences of being emotionally or sexually abused, or enmeshed by one or both parents. Intimacy has always seemed to create misery for you as an adult. But what you've been trying to avoid is enmeshment, not intimacy. Recovery includes (1) learning the difference between healthy intimacy and enmeshment, so you clearly see that intimacy is desirable and enhancing to your life; and (2) learning how to protect yourself with healthy boundaries from attempts at enmeshment by others.

1. Describe what you need to do to stop avoiding your relationships. (Give specific examples, such as, "Stop being away from the house every week night" or "Stop using arguments to control people," and so on.)

2. Examine your experience with the core symptoms of codependence, especially the symptoms regarding setting boundaries and acknowledging reality:

A. Write about experiences in childhood where caregivers did not have healthy boundaries, and so they enmeshed with you and violated your boundaries. Then write about how those experiences impact your adult life. (Use the form on the following page.)

Example

Instances in which my boundaries were transgressed in childhood	The impact of the boundary transgression on my adult life
My father was often physically abusive to me. He socked me in the arm with one knuckle or pinched me on the thigh until my eyes watered.	Today I really dislike it for anyone to touch me. Physical intimacy feels dangerous.

Instances in which my boundaries were transgressed in childhood	The impact of the boundary transgression on my adult life

B. Write about experiences in childhood in which your
caregiver used personal information about you to control
or manipulate you:

3. In the left column list the kinds of walls you have used in
order to avoid being known. In the right column write statements about how healthy boundaries will accomplish the
same protection with fewer harmful consequences to yourself
and the other person in your relationship:

Example

Walls used	How healthy boundaries can accomplish the same protection with fewer harmful consequences
Silence	With internal boundaries, I can give my preferences when my wife asks for them, and not feel guilty or ashamed if my wife doesn't like my preferences.

How healthy boundaries can accomplish the same protection with fewer harmful consequences	Walls used

4. In the left column of the form on the next page list things you are dealing with alone. In the right column write statements about how you might ask for support (sharing your experience so that someone else knows and cares) or help (asking for someone to do part of it for you or with you.)

Example

What I'm dealing with alone	How I might ask for support or help
My son, who lives with his mother, my first wife, steals money when he visits. I don't know what to do, but I sure get angry when I find the money missing.	I could tell my present wife what I suspect and the proof I have, and ask her to share ideas with me about what to do.
My boss reminds me of my father, and I have trouble getting along with him.	I could tell my wife about these feelings, telling her I just want her to listen and understand that this is a difficulty but I'm working on it. Or I could go to a counselor and discuss my problem with my boss and how he reminds me of my father.

How I might ask for support or help	What I'm dealing with alone

5. In the left column of the form on the next page list the ways you avoid being available to relate to people. In the right column write statements about ways you are willing to be involved with the person with whom you are in a close relationship.

Example

Ways I avoided being available for intimacy with a person in a relationship with me	Ways I am willing to be with a person in a relationship with me
Being away every night after work involved in volunteer work or drinking at the Pink Elephant.	Stay home two nights a week and be available for conversation with my children, to help with homework or talk, and to be available for conversation with my wife or to hear about her concerns with the checkbook.

Ways I am willing to be with a person in a relationship with me	Ways I avoided being available for intimacy with a person in a relationship with me

6. In the left column of the form on the next page list the ways you control the relationship. In the right column list statements about what you could do instead of the controlling behavior.

Example

Ways I controlled my relationship	What I could do instead of using this control method
Irritated argument.	Calmly state my position and listen courteously to the other person's point of view.
Harping about spending money.	Open a separate checking account for my wife out of which she spends money without answering to me.
Putting down my son for not being convincing in requests made to me.	Learn to say no without attacking him.

Ways I controlled my relationship	What I could do instead of using this control method

PERSONAL RECOVERY

If you have kept suffering through the emotional cycle created by being in a co-addicted relationship, either as a Love Addict or as a Love Avoidant, it may seem that there is little hope. But the four of us who have worked on this book want to testify that there is great hope.

As we've wrestled with this manuscript and thought back over our own difficulties with co-addicted relationships, we've been able to see how much recovery has taken place in our own close relating. We are all experiencing more serenity in relationships than we would have thought possible a few years ago. It has not been easy, and each of us has fallen back and had to begin again more than once. But the amazing good news is that we are much more aware. We manipulate and attack less often, which used to be our almost automatic and routine responses to people in our relationships. We find that with healthier boundaries we are less likely to react to our partners' behaviors as if we were puppets on a string. Instances of going into a life-long habit of emotional blast-off into orbits of pain and panic are fewer.

As we enjoy more and more the healthy characteristics of our relationships, and as we are able to give up some of our skewed, childish thinking about what to expect from those close to us, life has gotten much better. We are more comfortable negotiating differences, more able to see ourselves as having equal value in our relationships, and more able to make direct requests for intimacy and support.

It is our hope that this way of looking at the painful interactions between people in relationship can help you recognize and embrace the reality of the love addiction problem in your own life, bravely face the pain, and enter the process of recovery. We know now that the legacy we received from our childhood experiences of abandonment or enmeshment need not continue to rule our lives. There is a way out, as we and many others are now finding. It takes courage, trust, stamina, and a deep desire to walk out of the darkness of our current situations into a brighter day, a way of living that brings increased personal dignity, integrity, and inner serenity. And as we walk toward recovery, we can cease passing this painful legacy to our children.

One of the immature ideas that a childhood in a dysfunctional family can implant in our minds is the thought, "I can't stand this pain!" But that's just not true. We have found that with the help of a Higher Power, whom we call God, we *can* stand the pain of facing reality. What's more, this pain can be transformed into the birth pangs for a whole new experience of life and loving on the journey into recovery.

Welcome aboard!

A LOOK AT SOME OF THE PSYCHOLOGICAL LITERATURE REGARDING LOVE ADDICTION

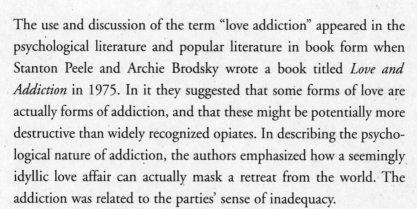

The use and discussion of the term "love addiction" appeared in the psychological literature and popular literature in book form when Stanton Peele and Archie Brodsky wrote a book titled *Love and Addiction* in 1975. In it they suggested that some forms of love are actually forms of addiction, and that these might be potentially more destructive than widely recognized opiates. In describing the psychological nature of addiction, the authors emphasized how a seemingly idyllic love affair can actually mask a retreat from the world. The addiction was related to the parties' sense of inadequacy.

In an earlier article in *Psychology Today,* Peele and Brodsky (1974) pointed out that Love Addicts might be people who need others to structure their life for them, and who cut themselves off from others and focus on developing relationships that are not growth inducing and are "nearly impossible to end."

Jane Simon (1975) discusses both healthy and neurotic aspects of love. She compares neurotic sexual attachments with drug addiction in terms of passivity, detachment, low self-esteem, and exploitation of others. She argues that healthy, mature love excludes mutual exploitation and promotes individual growth and self-fulfillment in both partners.

Seven years later Simon (1982) suggested that there are two types of love relationships: addictive and self-realizing. She discussed the developmental aspects in addictive relationships, sexual differences in such behavior, and the course of therapy in these cases.

Kerry Booth (1969) noted the need of male alcoholics to maintain a dependency status and avoid self-reliance.

Twenty years later Nadine Trocme, in *Psychologic Medicale* (1989), pointed out in treating alcoholics the patient's psychological dependence and avoidance of all objective relationships. The relevant point for *Facing Love Addiction* is that they reported a dysfunctionally dependent childhood relationship with the patient's mother that established a pattern of dependence repeated with the alcoholic's spouse and other important people in his or her life.

Back in 1981 Mary Hunter, *et al.* (1981) developed a "Love Scale" to measure love addiction. Another scale was developed by Australia's Judith Feeney and Patricia Noller (1990). This scale was to measure the "attachment style," attachment history, beliefs about relationships, self-esteem, limerance, loving, and love styles. Subjects who had childhood experiences of desertion or distance from a strong parent reported a lack of independence and a desire for a deep commitment in relationships. Analysis of the data indicated that attachment style is strongly related to self-esteem, and therefore to child-parent relationship history.

Dorothy Lewis, *et al.* (1991), in studying female delinquents, found that compared to a matched set of male delinquents, the females (having come from abusive households) often became enmeshed in violent relationships.

A. Charles-Nicolas, *et al.* (1989) explored possible childhood roots of adolescent and young adult drug addiction. Although they did not postulate any linear causal connection between traumatic events in drug addicts' childhoods and their current drug dependence, they found that addicts' inabilities to fully recall and elaborate such traumas induced them to resort to drugs rather than face them in their minds. They concluded that dysfunctional mother-infant relationships (for example, "fusion and/or rejections") appear to connect strongly with later substance dependence.

Grant Martin (1989) related the addictive model to marital affairs. He defines addiction as the progressive inability to start or stop an activity in spite of destructive consequences. Martin separates love addictions into three separate kinds (romance, relationships, and sexual), and presents characteristics and levels of each along with some suggestions for treatment.

Stanton Peele (1985) argued that the increasing recognition of the possibility of addiction to activities other than drug use seems to call for a reevaluation of key strands of thought about the nature of addiction—namely its relationship to the biological substratum and the relevance of cultural and individual interpretation of experience in addiction. He suggests requirements of a successful model of "pan-addiction."

Richard Miller (1987) presents a dialogue in which he questions pioneer Stanton Peele (1975) on the development of a unified theory of addiction, including a discussion of addictive behaviors, treatment of addiction, and addiction to experiences like love and stress as well as substances.

Thomas Timmreck (1990) discusses the literature on "love addiction" and provides some insights and therapeutic modalities, which he says have been effective for clients with love addiction.

In looking through the above psychological literature and then glancing at the Suggested Reading, it becomes apparent that almost

all of the literature about love addiction has been written in the past
ten years and that much of it is not related to what we are calling love
addiction. As we suggested in the preface, we are aware that we are
"writing ahead of the literature." The variables in what we are calling
love addiction or co-addicted relationships are numerous. And we are
relying primarily on Pia Mellody's clinical experience to describe the
painful, compulsive way of relating that we feel is crippling many
thousands of people who are baffled and confused about the intense
pain in their relationships.

References

Booth, Kerry G. (1969) *Dissertation Abstracts International*
30(4–8): 1893. Norman, OK: University of Oklahoma.

Charles-Nicolas, A., Voukassovitch, C., and Touzeau, D.
(March–April 1989) *Annales Medico-Psychologiques 147*(2): 241–44.

Feeney, Judith A. and Noller, Patricia. (February 1990) *Journal of
Personality and Social Psychology 58*(2): 281–91. Brisbane, Australia:
University of Queensland.

Hunter, Mary S., Nitschke, Cynthia, and Hogan, Linda (April
1981) *Psychological Reports 48*(2): 582. Arlington: University of Texas
Graduate School of Social Work.

Lewis, Dorothy O., Yeager, Catherine A., Cobham-Portorreal,
Celeste S., and Klein, Nancy, *et al.* (March 1991) *U.S. Journal of the
American Academy of Child and Adolescent Psychiatry 30*(2): 197–201.
New York: New York University Medical Center, Dept. of Psychiatry.

Martin, Grant L. (Winter 1989) *Journal of Psychology and
Christianity 8*(4): 5–25. Seattle, WA: CRISTA Counseling Service.

Miller, Richard E. (1987) *Employee Assistance Quarterly 3*(1):
35–56. Webster, NY: Xerox Health Management Program.

Peele, Stanton (March 1985) *British Journal of Addiction 80*(1): 23–25. Morristown, NJ: Human Resources Institute.

Peele, Stanton and Brodsky, Archie. *Love and Addiction* (Harvard: Harvard University Business School, 1975).

Peele, Stanton and Brodsky, Archie. (August 1974) *Psychology Today 8*(3): 22.

Simon, Jane. (Winter 1975) *American Journal of Psychoanalysis 35*(4): 359–64.

Simon, Jane. (Fall 1982) *American Journal of Psychoanalysis 42*(3): 253–63. New York: Institutes of Religion and Health.

Timmreck, Thomas C. (April 1990) *Psychological Reports 66*(2): 515–28. San Bernardino, CA: California State University.

Trocme, Nadine. (December 1989) *Psychologic Medicale 21*(14): 2143–46. Paris, France: Boucloaut Hospital, Internal Medicine Service.

SUGGESTED READING

Ackerman, Robert, and Susan Pickering. *Abused No More: Recovery for Women in Abusive and/or Codependent Alcoholic Relationships.* Blue Ridge Summit, PA: TAB Books, 1989.

Arterburn, Stephen. *Addicted to Love: Recovery from Unhealthy Dependency in Love, Romantic Relationships and Sex.* Ann Arbor, MI: Servant Publications, 1991.

Bireda, Martha. *Love Addiction: A Guide to Emotional Independence.* Oakland, CA: New Harbinger, 1990.

Covington, Stephanie. *Leaving the Enchanted Forest: The Path from Relationship Addiction.* San Francisco, CA: HarperSanFrancisco, 1988.

Cruse, Joseph. *Painful Affairs: Looking for Love Through Addiction and Codependency.* New York: Doubleday, 1989.

Diamond, Jed. *Looking for Love in All the Wrong Places: Overcoming Romantic and Sexual Addictions.* New York: Putnam Publishing Group, 1988 and 1989.

Firestone, Robert W., Ph.D. *The Fantasy Bond: Effects of Psychological Defenses on Interpersonal Relations.* New York: Human Sciences Press, Inc., 1987.

Gorski, Terence T. *The Players and Their Personalities: Understanding People Who Get Involved in Addictive Relationships.* Independence, MO: Herald House, 1989.

Grizzle, Ann. *Mothers Who Love Too Much: Breaking Dependent Love Patterns in Family Relationships.* Westminster, MD: Ivy Books, 1991.

Imbach, Jeff. *The Recovery of Love: Christian Mysticism and the Addictive Society.* New York: The Crossroad Publishing, 1991.

Kasl, Charlotte D. *Women, Sex, and Addiction: The Search for Love and Power.* San Francisco, CA: HarperSanFrancisco, 1990.

Lee, John H. *I Don't Want To Be Alone: For Men and Women Who Want to Heal Addictive Relationships.* Deerfield Beach, FL: Health Communications, 1990.

Lorrance, Laslow. *Love Addict at Eighty-Four: Confessions of an Old Romantic.* New York: Vantage, 1991.

May, Gerald G. *Addiction and Grace: Love & Spirituality in the Healing of Addictions.* San Francisco, CA: HarperSanFrancisco, 1991.

Mellody, Pia, and Andrea Wells Miller. *Breaking Free: A Workbook for Facing Codependence.* San Francisco, CA: HarperSanFrancisco, 1989.

Mellody, Pia, with Andrea Wells Miller and J. Keith Miller. *Facing Codependence: What It Is, Where It Comes From and How It Sabotages Your Life.* San Francisco, CA: HarperSanFrancisco, 1989.

Miller, Joy. *Addictive Relationships: Reclaiming Your Boundaries.* Deerfield Beach, FL: Health Communications, 1989.

Norwood, Robin. *Women Who Love Too Much.* New York: St. Martin's Press, 1985.

Norwood, Robin. *Letters from Women Who Love too Much: A Closer Look at Relationship Addiction and Recovery.* New York: St. Martin's Press, 1988.

Paul, Jordan and Margaret Paul. *From Conflict to Caring.* Minneapolis, MN: CompCare Publishers, 1988.

Peabody, Sue. *Addiction to Love.* Berkeley, CA: Ten Speed Press, 1989.

Peele, Stanton, and Archie Brodsky. *Love and Addiction.* New York: NAL-Dutton, 1976 and 1987.

Ricketson, Susan C. *Dilemma of Love: Healing Codependent Relationships at Different Stages of Life.* Deerfield Beach, FL: Health Communications, 1990.

Sandvig, Karen J. *Growing Out of An Alcoholic Family: Overcoming Addictive Patterns in Alcoholic Family Relationships.* Ventura, CA: Regal, 1990.

Schaef, Anne Wilson. *Escape from Intimacy: Untangling the "Love" Addictions: Sex, Romance, Relationships.* San Francisco, CA: HarperSanFrancisco, 1990.

Schaeffer, Brenda. *Is It Love or Is It Addiction?* San Francisco, CA: HarperSanFrancisco, 1987.

Weinhold, Barry. *Breaking Free of Addictive Family Relationships.* Dallas, TX: Stillpoint, 1991.

INDEX